IN PRAISE OF DR ALI AND INTEGRATED MEDICINE

"I am wholly convinced that the integrated health approach has the power to really make an immense difference to many people's lives... Dr Ali has done us a great service in pointing out the way forward during the coming century..." *H.R.H Prince of Wales*

"If Hippocrates had needed a doctor he would have sent for this man." *Selina Scott*

"Dr Ali's accurate diagnosis has always amazed me. His treatments always work." *Kate Moss*

"Dr Ali has saved me from pain – and from painkillers and their side-effects. Blessings on him." *Eve Arnold*

A remarkable self-help
programme to prevent and
treat all know back problems

Dr Ali's Ultimate Back Book

Dr Mosaraf Ali
with Ken Bridgewater

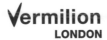
Vermilion
LONDON

1 3 5 7 9 10 8 6 4 2

Copyright © Dr Mosaraf Ali 2002

Dr Mosaraf Ali has asserted his right to be identified as the authors of this work in accordance with the Copyright, Designs and Patents Act 1988.

First published in 2002 by Vermilion,
an imprint of Ebury Press, Random House,
20 Vauxhall Bridge Road, London SW1V 2SA
www.randomhouse.co.uk

Random House Australia (Pty) Limited
20 Alfred Street, Milsons Point, Sydney,
New South Wales 2061, Australia

Random House New Zealand Limited
18 Poland Road, Glenfield, Auckland 10, New Zealand

Random House South Africa (Pty) Limited
Endulini, 5a Jubilee Road, Parktown 2193, South Africa

The Random House Group Limited Reg. No. 954009

Papers used by Vermilion are natural, recyclable products
made from wood grown in sustainable forests.

Typeset by seagulls
Text and cover design by The Senate
Printed and bound in GB by Scotprint Ltd, Haddington, East Lothian

A CIP catalogue record for this book is available from the British Library.

ISBN 0 09 188239 7

To Shahzad and Azeem

CONTENTS

ACKNOWLEDGEMENTS

This was not an easy book to write. How to condense over twenty years of experience and the observations derived from treating thousands of people with backache into a couple of hundred pages? Neither was the physical effort needed for treatment, such as massage and manipulation, easy. My body often ached – and the nights were often uncomfortable but I persevered in search of the truth about the way our bodies function or become ill.

I would like to thank all those patients who trusted me and tried my method even though it was sometimes painful. Although guided by my intuition, I was, in fact, trying a new concept of back pain management. In the initial phase of my work it was very much trial and error and sometimes I reverted back to methods such as acupuncture and anti-inflammatory medicines. I apologise to those whom I could not help.

My deep gratitude to Ken Bridgewater for his great patience in going through scribbled writings to catch grammatical and spelling errors, as they were mostly written between 3 a.m. and 6 a.m. He took great trouble in trying to prove logically my hypotheses in his own mind before allowing me to tell my readers about my findings. He tried to put his sleeping cat several times on a scale to see if it was heavier, but the creature woke up every time. Thus, we dropped my hypothesis that a dead body or a sleeping child or a paralysed person is heavier than normal. The concept of 'dead weight' could not be proved or disproved in this book.

I may be critical of the approach some of the osteopaths, physiotherapists, orthopaedic surgeons, and others, take in back pain management. For that, I deeply apologise. Perhaps my book will act as a guide to enhance their work to treat backache effectively, safely and cost-effectively.

I would like to also thank Ed Victor, my agent, everybody at Random House for their help, and Sue Peart and her team at YOU magazine for the serialisation of this book. Finally, I thank Colin Montgomerie for agreeing to write the foreword.

Dr Mosaraf Ali
London
www.dr-ali.co.uk

Foreword

I am privileged to write the foreword for *Dr Ali's Ultimate Back Book*, which I think is no less than a thesis, as it is based on his years of research and experience in the matter. The thousands of patients he has treated have given a deep insight into the cause and treatment of various types of backache.

The original idea that he has so beautifully elaborated in this book will no doubt make a lot of health professionals who manage backache think deeply about the role of muscles and one's well-being in its genesis.

Like his *Integrated Health Bible*, this book is so easy to read and understand. Knowing that people suffer from backache every day and are in great discomfort, I am sure this book will help people to understand their condition and help them to help themselves. These simple methods of treatment are easy to follow and they really do work.

My back is not only important to my general health but also crucial to the success of my career. I have experienced first hand the prowess Dr Ali has in this field and have benefited from his treatment enormously.

I wish Dr Ali a lot of success with this book and hope that he will continue to enlighten us with his original ideas, of which there are so many, in the future.

Colin Montgomerie

Introduction

The World Health Organisation has stated that low back pain costs Britain £6 billion per year (UK Clinical Standards Advisory Group,1994) and it costs the USA up to $85 billion per year (Frymoyer,1996). That's just low back pain. Add to that problems of the rest of the spine, particularly the neck, and the many conditions conventional medical science fails to relate to the spine and you have a sizable proportion of a national budget. Most of these conditions are preventable, almost certainly controllable and likely to be curable without drugs or surgery by Integrated Health, this being the culling of the best in all forms of medicine known to man.

Like almost any disease, however, a spine condition requires the co-operation of the patient if it is to be prevented, controlled or cured. This entails some understanding by the patient on how the back functions.

In this book I am going to introduce you to your back. In Part 1 I will show you how it is designed, how it is put together, how it works (as if it has a mind of its own), what are its weaknesses and how to look after it. In Part II, I will show you what can go wrong and how to put things right. Ultimately you have to decide what sort of a back you want to have and whether you want to stand upright in this world. Heaven forbid that you should wish to be regarded as spineless.

Please note that for Back oil, Lifestyle Massage oil and Joint oil please refer to www.dr-ali.co.uk or ring the Integrated Medical Centre on 020 7224 5111.

PART I

HOW THE
BACK WORKS

Chapter **1**

The Role of Muscles in Posture

Spine Design

Your spine is a tower. Let me ask you: would you say it was structured more like a tower of the Golden Gate Bridge or like the Eiffel Tower? Let's have a look at both and see if we can tell which is nearer.

The tower of a suspension bridge has massive cables attached to the top, one pulling it towards the land and the other towards the water. By their very nature they are both pulling down on the tower with enormous force. The tower is under massive compression. Fortunately, resisting compression is something concrete is particularly good at. The same effect happens to a tent pole, where the guy ropes, attached to the top to hold it up, tend to drive it into the ground.

The Eiffel Tower, on the other hand has no supporting cables. The steel network around its vertical axis is designed at every level just to hold up the weight and stresses of the structure above it and nothing more. The whole tower is under the least possible compression. It is significant that it is made of steel, not concrete.

Just for a moment imagine you are God, and you have observed that the precursor of man is starting to walk more and more upright, so his spine needs some redesign. Which model do you think you would choose? Would you put his new spine under great compression, squashing all the cushions between the vertebrae (the discs), or would you design it so the muscular cladding round the bones supported an upright posture, like the Eiffel Tower, without pulling down from the neck? This would ease all the vertebrae apart, making life as comfortable as possible for the discs.

Now these, as you have probably gathered, are very loaded questions. In fact conventional medical science would have us believe that huge back muscles, like the trapezius, stretching from the neck to far down the back, and the strong abdominal and chest muscles in the front, are the main means of keeping the posture of the back erect, pulling in both forward and backward directions to achieve postural balance and putting the discs under great compression. But as I am sure you worked out for yourself, that is not what one would expect from God or clever Nature. Surely one would expect the emphasis to be on the deep muscles and ligaments cladding the spine itself to hold it erect, putting minimum compression on the discs. If the discs do get compressed, it is much more likely that this is due to a sedentary lifestyle, withering the deep cladding muscles, against Nature's intent, than to a monumental blunder by God.

This is so fundamental to our treatment of our spines that I am now going to gather what evidence there is to show us which way God designed our backs.

Gaining Evidence

First let's try an imaginary experiment. Take a long sausage balloon and instead of blowing air in it, fill it up with a dozen or so glass marbles. If you now lay it on the table the marbles will tend to stay in a line because the rubber sheath forms a sort of ligament around them. However, if you pick the sausage up and try and make it stand vertically, it will flop over. It cannot stand up on its own because of the weight of the marbles. Now put your two fists around the sausage, one above the other, and, of course, you can make the string of marbles stand up, held vertical by the muscles in the palms of your hands. Indeed, if you squeeze with your palms, the sausage will elongate as the pressure of your palms separate the marbles from each other. There are no cables or guy ropes at the top, the muscles in your hands are providing all the uplift necessary to keep the string of marbles upright, which are under no compression. Your palms have provided an anti-gravitational force counteracting the weight of the marbles.

So it is with your spine. Strip all the muscles off the vertebrae and the skeleton will collapse. It is the muscles, not just the bones, that keep you erect.

Can a child in deep sleep be made to sit up on a chair? Can a totally paralysed person be made to sit or stand without support?

You tell me – but the marbles wouldn't stand up without muscles, would they?

Why then has medicine, which regards the skeleton as the stable structure of the body, not considered that in fact muscles create the key force, in an alert or toned-up state, that support our erect posture? Remove the nervous impulse that tones up muscles and makes them contract, and the muscles will become flaccid and inert resulting in the collapse of the body. Tranquillise an elephant and it collapses.

Role of Muscles

In case you are not sure about certain anatomical terms, I will try to explain them as I go along, but just for a start:

- a muscle is a piece of meat, full of blood;
- a tendon is an enormously strong white fibrous tissue, like flexible steel, that joins a muscle to a bone;
- a ligament is the gristle surrounding joints that keeps the ends of the bones in place.

You can see all three very clearly in a turkey leg. You eat the meat, but there is no way you can eat the tendons or the ligaments – you give them to the dog.

Without the muscles and their tendons, the skeletal system is useless on its own. The main function of the bones is to provide stability and hard surfaces to which muscles can be attached. The bones therefore play a secondary, not a primary role in movement and posture maintenance. Muscles with their tone or fitness create an anti-gravitational force that keeps Homo Sapiens erect. The skeletal system, especially the spine, without its muscles can hardly stand up on its own. It certainly can't support the weight of the heart, lungs, liver, intestines, kidneys etc without collapsing. Only the spinal muscles can create that force to keep the spine erect. The same principles apply to the legs and hips, and without their musculature they would not be able to support the weight of the torso and the head.

When Muscles Are Inactive

As you go to sleep in a chair, the neck is the first to give in and your head flops over, at first jerking up in starts but, as sleep deepens, the back also loses power. Even with the best of intentions, a person in deep sleep cannot stay erect. The neck muscles become so flaccid that they cannot even keep the head in the central balanced position when reclined. That is why some airlines' executive class seats have flexible 'wings' on either side of the head so that it does not loll to one side or the other causing neck tension and muscle spasm.

A sleeping child seems extra heavy to carry and every parent who has ever transferred a child from a car or sofa knows the difference in lift. The same child when awake apparently weighs much less, because its muscles are alive and active. Doctors and nurses transferring paralysed, comatose and dead patients from the bed to the trolley know very well how heavy the person feels. The term 'deadweight' is derived from this phenomenon.

Patients who have been bedridden for a long time find it extremely difficult to walk as their muscles are unfit, though the bones haven't changed, and the body feels heavier in the first couple of days. As the muscle tone builds up the movement becomes easier.

So it is clear that muscles, rather than bones, control our posture.

Muscle Fitness

Those who exercise and are physically fit often have bulky muscles but they are generally fairly agile. Unfit and tired people have extremely sluggish bodies and have greater inertia than normal people. Boxers, sprinters, gymnasts, dancers and the like are so agile and quick in their movements because their muscle tone is perfectly balanced. Ballerinas with a well-balanced weight and muscle tone are free in their movements. They are 'as light as a feather' and they can be lifted and moved with ease and grace. Martial arts practitioners, having concentrated on building muscle tone, can perform their swift and almost acrobatic movements with perfection and ease.

So it is the fitness of the muscles that displays our well-being.

Nobody has ever 'scientifically' studied or proved the extent to which muscles support our body weight and whether it is they that carry the weight of the body and not the spine. The conclusions that I have drawn are based on logic. Although scientific proof, based on mathematical, physical or chemical analysis, can be very accurate in some matters, it is inadequate in solving the mysteries of Nature, of which the human body is only a part, and helpless when it comes to studying Nature's laws and phenomena. Ancient scientists and philosophers used logic to prove their point. They were often backed up by human experience or simple experiment. Modern science considers these methods too primitive or 'subjective' for any validation and tends to reject them outright. They want 'evidence-based medicine'.

So to analyse our spine design we need logic, not science.

In the following chapters, as you have probably guessed, I will show that logic leads us to the conclusion that it is the muscles closely cladding the spine that keeps it erect, muscles that are unfortunately so inaccessible that only special exercises and massage can keep them fit. The exercises recommended by books and gymnasia tend to tone up the greater superficial muscles, important in bending and lifting, but are only of secondary significance in posture and disc protection. Thus science has misled us and fitness instruction tends to be misguided.

Genesis of Back Problems

In the later chapters, I will also try to explain with logic and personal experience the true origin of disc problems, backache and postural troubles using the concept that muscles, and particular muscles at that, play the primary role in the prevention and genesis of spine problems. The bones, and even the bending and lifting muscles, play only an inconsequential part in these problems. Except in the case of direct trauma or injury, the problems of joints, discs and other bone-like structures predominantly result from weakness or defect of the spinal and related muscles. I will show that the spine needs very special treatment to remain healthy, but with Integrated Health it can normally remain so for life.

Treatment of Back Problems

With our normal lifestyle, however, things do go wrong. Medicine has led us to believe that back problems originate from the vertebral joints (facet joints) and from discs and their related complications. They say the discs degenerate because of wear and tear, lack of exercise and traumas. Backaches are therefore referred on to orthopaedic surgeons, who either operate or refer patients to related specialists. The entire spine is treated by orthopaedic surgeons if the bones or joints are involved, or by neurologists and neurosurgeons if the nerves (irritation by discs) are involved. If muscles and inflammation of joints are suspected, physiotherapists are involved. If the spine has impacted the circulatory system, however, the case should be (but rarely is) referred to a cardiologist, immunologist or psychiatrist, as such a concept is completely outside the purview of the orthopaedic surgeon. Dr Hamilton Hall, an internationally established back specialist in Toronto, defined an orthopaedic surgeon on page 1 of his famous book *The Back Doctor* as a bone and joint doctor. Need I say more?

An English girl, **Betty,** was taken to the Accident and Emergency Department in a leading hospital in a Commonwealth country with severe spinal spasms and pain. Her condition was diagnosed as a 'Slipped Disc'. She was admitted and put on traction. Later she was taken to physiotherapy during which a knee was dislocated. The orthopaedic surgeon said the tendons of the knee were too slack and had to be tightened. He performed the operation. Two days later he apologised to the girl's parents for having operated on the wrong knee and with their permission repeated the operation on the other leg. The screw he had put in the first knee soon came loose and a third operation had to be performed. Betty was in the hospital for five months, after which she went back to England to recuperate. Here her condition was diagnosed by an immunologist as Systemic Lupus Erythmatosis (SLE), an autoimmune disease that can affect the joints. She has been registered as physically disabled for the last 20 years and spends much of her time in a wheelchair. It turned out to be a case of a wrong referral presenting the orthopaedic surgeon with a problem outside his purview.

Treatment of Muscles

In general, physiotherapists without special postgraduate training act as 'para-medics', equivalent to nurses who help medics to carry out some of their labour-intensive jobs, except that they function quite independently. Some doctors have only a vague idea of what goes on in the physiotherapy department. Thus there is no strong rapport between doctors and physiotherapists.

Choice of Practitioner

Physiotherapists look at backache generally as a problem related to the vertebral column. Muscles, in the opinion of most physiotherapists, play a secondary role. That is why traction, electric currents, heat etc are predominantly used to treat backaches. Some general back-strengthening exercises and remedial massages are also used, but they tend to focus on the large superficial muscles (the ones you can massage directly) rather than on the deep spine-supporting muscles. The fact that traction is used to release pressure on the nerves (and incidentally allow the deep spinal muscles to wither and ligaments to tear) is definite proof that they look at backache primarily as a mechanical problem. Belts and lumbar supports are also recommended along those very principles of mechanical cause of backache. They are very successful in treating patients with acute (sudden/severe) conditions but fail miserably to treat chronic (persistent) backache and prevent it. The fact that an acute backache becomes chronic after a few weeks indicates that physiotherapy is unable to manage or cure it and that such an approach towards the treatment of this condition has some fundamental flaws. What cannot cure a disease in an acute stage will not be able to cure it in its chronic stage. The first stage gradually moves into the second when its course is not checked by treatment. There is no evidence for the principle that longer and more intensive treatment will cure a disease in its chronic stage. The fact that a disease has become chronic shows that the treatment has not worked.

The bulk of the body consists of muscles (meat) and yet conventional medicine has made little or no effort to study their role and functions. Myology (myos – muscles, logos – study or knowledge) assists in muscular diagnosis, and neurology, which treats muscles and nerves as one, treats neuro-muscular disabilities such as polio, stroke, cerebral palsy, multiple sclerosis with the help of physiotherapists. In conventional medicine, therefore, there is no therapeutic speciality for muscular disorders other than myology, which investigates muscles through biopsy and electrophysiological studies.

In recent years, however, sports medicine has grown up to meet the demand for stamina, endurance, fitness and treatment of sports-related medical problems. Thus muscles became the primary target for investigation and study in sports medicine. Besides muscles, sports medicine studies nutritional, psychological and cardiovascular aspects of sports. The link with the rest of the body is beginning to appear.

Sports injuries are treated by physiotherapists, however, just like any other form of disease of the muscles, bones, joints and ligaments. It is part of a rehabilitation and anti-inflammatory treatment plan. Some physiotherapists working in this area may specialise in muscle-building programmes but generally it is the fitness instructors who actually specialise in exercises and muscle-building.

Introducing Integrated Medicine

I have researched back problems for over 20 years, making extensive comparisons of thousands of patient records. Because medical science and procedures for the spine are so inadequate and misleading I have found it necessary to go back to first principles. 2,500 years ago in Greece Hippocrates, the father of medicine, advocated what he called 'Regimen Therapy', which boosted the body's own healing power, based on diet, exercises and massage. He said people would not be ill if they ate well, did regular exercises and had periodic massage to alleviate stress and strain, while in sickness the same procedures led to more rapid recovery. I have made this my basic principle in my work in Integrated Health. Massage in particular creates a sense of well-being and invigorates the body by removing aches and improving blood circulation. After Hippocrates, the Romans perpetuated this, especially in their public baths, as did the great Persian physician Avicenna, a thousand years later. By working on muscles, passively by massage and actively through exercises, it is possible to release additional energy required when a person is being healed or treated. Ask any fatigued or stressed person how he or she feels after a session of good therapeutic massage and the answer will invariably be 'excellent'.

Regrettably, massages were gradually excluded from Western medicine until quite recently, when sports medicine rediscovered their effectiveness.

In the Orient, however, muscle therapies remain intact today, in literally every country or region. They realise that muscles not only help us to remain erect, move, carry out physical work etc, but also have reserves of vital energy, which can be enhanced by exercises such as 'Chi' in China and 'Prana' in India. In these regions, latent energy is recycled by physical massage in order to create a feeling of well-being.

Interestingly, this logical philosophy can be supported by science. The majority of the ATP or energy molecules, required for all chemical action in the body, are synthesised in the mitochondria (power stations) of the muscle fibres. Releasing these ATP molecules into the bloodstream can be expected to increase the energy available for the body to give itself a boost. So the ancient medical men were on to a scientific truth after all.

Here are some examples of massages used in different countries:

Shiatsu

A Japanese style of massage using point-pressure technique, stretching with soft- and hard-tissue manipulation.

Abhyanga

Part of traditional Indian Ayurvedic treatment called 'Panchakarma'. It is performed with medicated oils which are massaged into the body and then squeezed out as if to eliminate the absorbed oil along with the body toxins.

Thai massage

This technique combines deep pressure on muscles and ligaments with manipulation of bones and soft tissues. It stretches muscles and restores normal blood flow into them.

Marma

This is an ancient Indian form of martial arts. The Marma massage involves stimulation of Marma (trigger) points, stretching of muscles and tendons and gentle manipulation of the spine.

Acupressure

This Chinese system of massage of the pressure points in the body, is used as an alternative to acupuncture. The so-called Meridians are also massaged. Toi Na or push-pull massage is another form used in traditional Chinese medicine.

Bomo Massage

The Bomos are traditional healers in Malaysia and Indonesia. They use coins to apply deep pressure on the skin and muscles, often causing bruising. This is a painful procedure but it stimulates and tones up muscles, invigorating the body's energy system.

Swedish Massage

This is a gentle massage of the skin and superficial muscles, basically designed to improve circulation and remove fatigue.

Bear Massage

In Turkey bears used to be trained to walk over the back of a patient.

Vacuum Massage

In Russia a cup connected to an apparatus that compresses and rarifies air alternately. This cup is rubbed along muscles to vibrate them with air (suction and release).

Indian Dai Massage

Used for mother and child for 40 days after the delivery to help the mother recuperate, remove excess fat and stretch marks and to help the newborn to recover from the physical and mental trauma of birth.

Exercises

Besides these passive treatments of muscles, there are also systems of exercises in different countries to tone up muscles and invigorate them. Thus there is yoga in India, tai chi in China, gymnastics, aerobics, martial arts (Marma, judo, wrestling), sports, athletics, swimming etc. These are designed to improve the cardiovascular system, tone up muscles, build stamina and endurance, release physical and mental stress and invigorate the body. Exercises are crucial in a person's life for maintaining general health.

The growth of the culture of massage in the West in recent years and the practice of various specific exercises like yoga, Pilates, tai chi etc, has shown positive results in stress management and well-being. Although aromatherapy, using aromatic oils as the main therapeutic component of a gentle stroking massage, is the most popular method of complementary medical therapy, other muscle-orientated therapies like deep-tissue massage, sports massage, Shiatsu etc are growing very quickly. Many mainstream hospitals allow massage as a form of relaxing and invigorating therapy. The Royal Marsden Hospital, the leading cancer centre in the UK, has an aromatherapist visiting patients who are going through heavy treatments like chemotherapy and radiotherapy.

Impact of Muscles on Health

We can now clearly see why muscles are so important to the body. Whether conventional medical science recognises the role fully or not is a different issue, but practice and common sense shows that their role is vital to the well-being of the body. They build and store energy (in the form of glycogen complex sugar molecules), carry out locomotion (movement) and physical activities, and above all maintain the body's erect posture.

According to ancient yogic principles, the four parameters of good health are:

1

good appetite

2

proper elimination (of waste products)

3

sound sleep

4

erect posture

If the spine is straight it keeps the nerves free from compression, nerves that control movement, sense pain and also carry out involuntary functions like heartbeat, breathing, digestion etc. These autonomous (involuntary) nerve fibres also emerge from the spinal cord. Therefore, the spine contains local control centres of the body's various functions. An erect spine is not only the sign of good health but also of well-being. Tired and sick people look bent over and have a bad physical posture. The cervical spine in the neck also contains and protects the vertebral arteries that feed the subconscious brain. Neck conditions can therefore interfere with the circulation to that most vital part of the body and contribute to psychological and other often surprising problems, which I discuss in Chapter 12.

Muscles and Posture

An erect posture is maintained by spinal, abdominal, leg and other supportive muscles. In fact the entire musculature of the body participates in maintaining the body's posture in some way or the other. We will see in the following chapter how exactly this is carried out. The weight-bearing function of the various muscles determines the state of the joints, discs, bones etc. The wear and tear of these structures depend on how well the muscles carry the body's weight in rest, stress, exercises and at work. The integrity of the spine, in its influence on nerves and blood vessels, determines the performance of every system of the body. Only if we accept this will it become clear how much we depend upon our backs, and the extent to which we need a gatekeeper, or complete General Practitioner, to guide us to the right specialist. Conventional medicine, represented by orthopaedic surgeons in matters of back problems, seems to think that discs and joints are the root cause of most back-related problems and that such problems are confined to the back. We will argue and logically try to prove that this concept is a long way from the truth. But first let us consider how muscles work.

Chapter 2

How Muscles Work

Essential for Health

Life without muscles would not be possible. Heartbeat, blood circulation, digestion, elimination, sweating, breathing, chewing, vision, movement etc are all controlled by various types of muscle. Basically there are three types of muscle:

1

Skeletal muscles, the voluntary muscles connected to the skeletal system

2

Smooth muscles or involuntary muscles like the muscles of bladder, gut, blood vessels etc, and

3

Cardiac or heart muscles.

The skeletal muscles are very complex in their structure. The Figure on page 17 shows how they are subdivided into various units. The smallest units of muscles consist of thin and thick filaments made up of protein chains, actin and myosin respectively. These filaments cluster together in the sarcomere (sarcos – flesh, mere – part). These sarcomeres bundle together to form myofibril (myos – muscles, *fibrillae* – small fibres) which in turn form muscle fibre. A group of muscle fibres form muscle fascicle, which are units of skeletal muscles. So the progression is: protein chains – filaments – sarcomeres – myofibril – muscle fibres – fascicle – units of skeletal muscles.

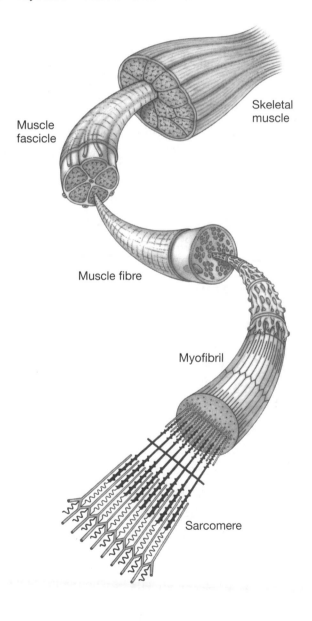

Skeletal muscle

Muscle fascicle

Muscle fibre

Myofibril

Sarcomere

Need for Energy

One of the main characteristics of muscles is that they have a rich network of blood vessels, supplying nutrients and oxygen and removing waste products. Muscle contraction, producing tension or pull, is an active process, requiring energy. The shortening of the length of muscles is brought about by the protein of sarcomeres (actin, myosin) interweaving, like the 'teeth' of two combs sliding into each other. This tension/shortening pulls bones, the surfaces on which the tendons of muscles are attached, and causes movements.

Some motor units within any particular muscle are always active, even when the muscle is not contracting. The contractions of these muscle fibres do not produce enough tension to cause movement but they do tense and firm up muscles. This resting tension in a skeletal muscle is called muscle tone. Lack of muscle tone can make a muscle look limp and flaccid, whereas even with the slightest tone the muscles become alert. It is muscle tone that makes the biceps look as they are, even when they are not contracting. Muscle shapes are produced by muscle tone even in the resting position when most muscle fibres relax. Resting muscle tone stabilises bones and joints, while lack of it can allow a joint to collapse. For example, stroke victims with loss of muscle power in one arm often have the shoulder joint dislocated with the weight of the arm. The deltoid (around the shoulder joint) muscles are so flaccid that they cannot keep the head of the humerus bone fixed into the socket of the shoulder joint.

Muscle tone also helps to act as a shock absorber that cushions the impact of a sudden bump or shock. A strong muscle tone is essential for preparedness for sports and exercises where sudden movements happen. Exercises also build up muscle tone.

Contraction

There are two known types of muscle contractions – isotonic and isometric. In isotonic contraction (iso – equal, tonus – tension) the length of the muscles change while the tension inside and outside remains constant. Lifting an object off the floor, walking, jogging etc are isotonic contractions. In isometric (iso – equal, metric – measure), the muscle as a whole does not change its length and yet it is contracted to its full capacity. Examples are pushing an immovable object (e.g. a wall), trying unsuccessfully to pick up a heavy object, resistance exercises etc.

Energy supply

Contraction of muscles needs phenomenal amounts of energy and therefore, in muscles, one sees a system of energy molecule production which appears nowhere else. Active muscle cells have myoglobin, which is similar to haemoglobin in blood, and this has the capability of absorbing oxygen and storing it as reserve. That is why skeletal muscles that are very active are red in colour like blood. Besides this, the muscle fibres have numerous mitochondria ('power stations') that produce energy molecules or ATP (Adenosine Triphosphates) through aerobic or oxygen-consuming conversion of glucose. Even this often does not produce enough energy to meet the demand, so muscles are gifted by Nature with two other physiological characteristics:

1

The ability to store glucose in the form of glycogen, which can be broken up as and when energy demand arises, and

2

The ability to carry out anaerobic (without oxygen) burning of glucose into energy molecules and lactic acid.

Thus we see that Nature has given skeletal muscles some unusual capacity to generate their own energy without depending on the liver and other organs to send the surplus. Skeletal muscles:

a

have their own oxygen-binding protein (myoglobin)

b

can carry out both aerobic and anaerobic types of glucose breakup to generate energy

c

store glycogen (glucose compound)

d

have a rich network of blood vessels to supply glucose and calcium, which is absolutely vital to the proteins of muscles as they cannot shorten or shrink without these nutrients, as well as remove waste products like carbon dioxide.

Contraction of muscles creates oxygen demand in the entire body, as its own system takes up most of the oxygen from the blood. The body then increases the heart rate and breathing to meet the demand. That is why the breathing is faster and the pulse rate goes up while running or doing strenuous exercises. Even when exercising stops, the breathing and heart rate continue to be high for some time to meet the demand. Exercising is the only natural way to:

a

improve circulation

b

make the heart pump more and improve its own muscle tone

c

increase energy reserves in the body

d

burn excess fat and sugar deposits or reserve in the body

e

tone up the muscles in the body to create a feeling of general well-being.

Excessive Use of Energy

The only undesirable complication of excessive skeletal muscle contractions or exercise is that it results in the accumulation of lactic acid in muscles. Normally glucose is converted to carbon dioxide and water in the mitochondria using oxygen molecules (see page 19). When the muscles are very active, these mitochondria cannot work fast enough to meet the demand for energy molecules, and so the muscle tissue releases energy molecules by anaerobic (without oxygen) conversion of glucose into lactic acid and energy molecules. If the demand for energy molecules persists and the mitochondria cannot meet the demand because of inadequate oxygen supply the level of lactic acid rises. This results in changing the chemistry of muscle fibres and they stop contracting till the demand for oxygen supply is met and the mitochondria are able to convert lactic acid quickly into carbon dioxide and water. This by-product of incomplete combustion of glucose, lactic acid, is generally harmful to the body especially the heart tissue. Besides producing cramps, stiffness and aches in muscles, it slows down muscle function in general, leading to fatigue. The lactic acid level of blood is frequently checked in sportsmen during training to assess the state of muscle functioning and fitness.

Fatigue

Muscle fatigue is a state in which muscle fibres can no longer contract. Its main cause is accumulation of lactic acid in muscles, which inhibits their contractile function. This is Nature's own way of applying brakes to the desire to do more. Marathon runners give up as they go along, especially if they are not adequately trained, and not all will reach the final destination. Muscle fatigue gives the muscles a chance to replenish the energy reserve and to remove waste products. All physical activities produce some degree of fatigue. Smaller muscles like the eye muscles and the muscles of the hand get fatigued more easily. Those who have written for long periods of time know very well that after a while their muscles become so fatigued that they cannot function any more. Children during tests or exams often write fast and experience fatigue, pain and inability to write after a while. They are compelled to stop.

Need for rest

Thus one must balance the period of work and rest. Nature gave us sleep precisely for this reason, so that muscles can replenish their energy, carry out the repair work of wear and tear and remove waste products and lactic acid. If we don't sleep enough and work very hard and dig into the time reserved for recuperation, the muscles will give in and create exhaustion. Even with the best of intention and mental stamina, the muscles will not function with the same ability. Sportsmen are advised to sleep or rest before a big event.

Muscle Performance

Muscle performance is characterised by *power*, the maximum tension an individual muscle or a group of muscles can produce, and *endurance*, the amount of timefor which an individual can perform that activity. Two major factors determine muscle performance: the types of muscle fibres involved and physical conditioning and training.

Types of muscle fibre

There are three major types of skeletal muscle fibres, known to myologists, in the human body: fast (twitching), slow (twitching) and intermediate (twitching) fibres.

Fast fibres

constitute the vast majority of skeletal muscle and they acquire their name from the fact that they can twitch, or contract-and-relax, very soon after stimulation (in approximately a 100th of a second). They are large in diameter, contain densely packed myofibrids, have large glycogen (stored glucose) reserves and relatively less myoglobin and fewer mitochondria. They are geared up for immediate and quick action. They do not have the time to wait for slow blood flow and therefore have very few capillaries. These muscles produce powerful and quick contractions and therefore have no time or capability for utilising oxygen to produce energy molecules (thus less blood flow, fewer mitochondria, less myoglobin). They use the quick and convenient anaerobic path of glucose utilisation, thus producing more lactic acid as a by-product. This is why fast muscle fibres fatigue so easily. They do their job and fag out. A sprinter dashes for the 100m race and almost collapses at the end as he or she is barely able to stand for a few minutes. Ask them to run another race shortly afterwards and the result will be very poor performance. Poorly trained runners get 'a stitch' – a spasm with pain. These muscles have no endurance to match other types of muscle fibres. As they have poor blood supply and less myoglobin, they are pale in colour.

Slow fibres

are only half the diameter of fast ones and take almost three times as long to contract after stimulation, but they can remain contracted for a longer period of time. These muscle fibres have myoglobin, a dense network of capillaries, many mitochondria and have smaller glycogen reserves (that is why they are not bulky muscles). These muscle fibres use other sources of energy as well, such as carbohydrates (amino acids, fatty acids). The muscles have less power but more endurance and, as they use aerobic utilisation of glucose to generate the moderate demand for energy molecules, they do not fatigue so easily. The rich blood supply ensures that the oxygen demand is met and the waste products are removed adequately to maintain the contractions of these muscle fibres. Slow fibres are responsible for posture (sitting, standing) and can remain contracted for a long period of time without getting fatigued. As these muscle fibres have myoglobin and a rich network of blood capillaries, they are dark red in colour (true red meat).

Intermediate fibres

have properties intermediate between those of fast and slow muscle fibres. They have more endurance than fast muscle fibres and more power that slow muscle fibres. Marathon runners train to develop this type of muscle as they have power as well as endurance.

Muscle training

One type of muscle can transform itself into another type through training. Weightlifters and bodybuilders can build up intermediate muscle fibres from fast-twitching biceps and other muscles. The proportion of different muscle fibres in a group of muscles can change according to the training that they undergo. The proportion of fast and slow muscle fibres is genetically determined but the proportion of intermediate muscle fibres to fast fibres can increase due to athletic training.

In humans most muscle fibres are mixed and therefore appear pink. The back and calf muscles are dominated by slow muscle fibres and are therefore red in colour and they maintain posture. Eye and hand muscles, which carry out brisk movements, are white in colour as they contain fewer blood vessels and less myoglobin.

Repeated muscle training leads to the development of more mitochondria, larger glycogen reserves and a higher concentration of enzymes and proteins in muscles. All these increase the muscle bulk in general and muscles get hypertrophied or bulky. The number of muscle fibres does not change as that is genetically determined, but their contents (proteins, glycogen, enzymes, mitochondria) may change. Some people remain skinny no matter how much they exercise or how much they eat. Their muscle bulk may marginally improve. This is due to an individual's constitution. Sumo wrestlers build up huge muscle bulk and fat reserves through training and diet.

When I was a student in the former Soviet Union, I came to know through my professor in physiology that Soviet sportsmen drank *keffir*, an especially prepared bacterial yoghurt drink which provided amino acid chains to build up protein in muscles. They also took ginseng (Siberian) to improve muscle power and endurance. That is why the Soviet weightlifters and other sportsmen were unbeatable at the Olympics.

Some sportsmen used steroids or testosterone to build up muscles. These drugs increase muscle bulk only when the muscles are exercised and so there is no easy way of building up muscle bulk. There is no proven benefit of this artificial use of muscle bulk enhancers but their harmful effects are well recorded.

Muscles can atrophy too when not used so frequently. They lose their bulk. This is clearly noted when a leg or foot is put in a cast after a fracture. Some conditions like polio affect the nerves and therefore cause paralysis and atrophy of muscles in the legs and other affected limbs.

Summary

Thus, to summarise, we could say that scientists have found out the following facts about muscles:

1

There are three types of muscle – skeletal, smooth and cardiac

2

Skeletal muscles are generally voluntary and can be made to contract at will

3

Smooth muscles are involuntary and cannot be controlled by the conscious brain (walls of blood vessels, bladder, and gut etc)

4

Skeletal muscles are subdivided into three types of muscle fibres:

a fast fibres, containing less blood and myoglobin, pale in colour and carrying out sudden and brisk movements. They fatigue easily.

b slow fibres, containing dense blood vessels, mitochondria and ample myoglobin, red in colour and carrying out slow and prolonged movements like maintaining posture. They do not fatigue so easily.

c intermediate fibres are in between fast and slow fibres. They do not fatigue as easily as fast fibres (like posture-maintaining muscles).

5

Muscle contraction is either:

a isometric, where the length of muscles does not change.

b isotonic, where the tone in muscles does not change but the length changes (as in movements).

6

Muscles consume a huge amount of energy when contracting and therefore have to generate their own energy molecules. These are produced by:

a aerobic methods in slow fibres, as oxygen is readily available from blood and myoglobin

b anaerobic methods in fast fibres where energy molecules are produced by incomplete combustion of glucose without using oxygen. This latter method produces more lactic acid, which is the origin of muscle fatigue.

7

Muscles contract because of stimulation by motor nerves of the fibres, which in turn, through a complex biochemical reaction in the presence of calcium, produce a sliding of specialised protein fibres into each other, causing contraction. Thus muscles have neurological as well as physical aspects of their function. They conduct electrical impulses as well as generate tension or power through actual physical movement.

Chapter 3

The Great Blunder

Flaws in Physiology

Myology, a branch of neurology, is the science that studied the skeletal muscles and their functions very meticulously. Thus the contents of muscles with their structures, like specialised blood and lymph supply, myoglobin, mitochondria, nerve fibres etc are very well known. The fact that muscles have protein strains that slide into each other to produce contraction or shortening of length is unique to this tissue.

The physiology (study of the functions) of muscles, which is a very complex matter, has been thorough but not without flaws. It has left many questions unanswered. Somehow, the existing tools used to study muscle function are not adequate to study living tissue. Unfortunately science has used its own limited methods and studied muscles as if they were like elastic bands that responded to electrical currents. Nature is much more complex than that and its laws are even more complicated. For the moment logic and not electrophysiology would be a better method to study living tissue like muscles. I am sure that one day there will be advanced ways of analysis that will give us better clues about the way life processes function, but until then some old-fashioned methods like logic and common sense may be more effective in the explanations.

Sports Science Breakthrough

Sometimes, observation of simple phenomena in living tissue can give important clues about its function. For example Soviet sports scientists, determined to thrust their own athletes ahead of the West in a one-upmanship war, discovered that skeletal muscles have their own pumping mechanism. It stemmed from a simple logical question: how do skeletal muscles supply blood to their own tissue in a heavily contracted state? The contracted muscles would offer such a powerful resistance that no fluid could ever pass through them. It seems an impossible task and yet, in the working state, muscle fibres need all the energy there is to maintain the supply and somehow they get it. Anaerobic breakdown of sugar – glycolysis – is one way of doing it without using oxygen or blood, but that is not enough as the demand for energy is huge.

A simple observation made by sports scientists of the muscle tissue gave them the clue. When weightlifters picked the weight up and held it above their heads for a few seconds in that position to register their success, their arm muscles began to vibrate and shake in a rhythmic pattern. The heavy weight (sometimes 250 lbs of it) was supported by muscles and the energy demand was phenomenal. To meet this demand muscles relaxed and became taut again in quick succession, thus acting like a pump to allow the exchange of blood and fluids. Thus a new phenomenon or functional property of skeletal muscles was discovered, namely that muscles have their own pumping mechanism.

In the case of weightlifters, it was obvious to the onlookers that their arm muscles shook rhythmically at peak performance. Soviet scientists began to study this phenomenon and made a gadget that applied low-level electric currents to mimic the pumping mechanism using the same rhythm. This shortened the recovery period of fatigued muscles. The performance of Soviet sportsmen automatically improved with this technique. This was often used to treat the muscles of ballerinas in between strenuous acts so that muscles would be instantly invigorated to produce one stunning performance after another.

Similarly, it has been noticed that a simple massage of the most active muscles recycles the blood and reinstates their functions in full, even after intensive training. Although science could not find any explanation for it initially, it is used widely in sports medicine and those who deal with fitness and performance have made massage into an essential part of the sportsmen's routine rituals. Sports teams have trained physical therapists or masseurs who routinely use massage to treat and maintain the vigour of muscles. All this came about from the observation of several oriental methods of muscle treatment.

The biggest mistake medical science has made is in classifying weight-bearing muscles under the heading of voluntary skeletal muscles. This blunder has led to a series of other mistakes that has brought great confusion in understanding a common problem like backache. It is almost like telling the first lie and then following it by a series of lies to cover up the original. A single mistake has led to frequent mistakes in diagnosis, management and prevention of backaches.

Here is how it all started.

The early physiologists studying muscles began by concentrating on the neuro-mechanical aspects of their functions. Muscles were compared to nerves as they conducted electric current across their membranes just like nerves. Muscles and nerves are the only groups of tissue that respond to electrical stimuli and produce their own potential. Their membranes are charged and are very receptive to electrical impulses from other nerves endings. Muscle cells obviously have an additional quality and that is their contractibility. Thus the electrical nature of muscles allows them to spread 'messages' quickly across their entire length (sometimes muscle cells can be as long as the entire muscle) and facilitate contraction uniformly. No other form of message can be transmitted so quickly, given the existing resistance (of fluids, proteins).

Looking in the Wrong Place

Medical science also focused on the biochemical nature of muscles. They found that myo-filaments, the smallest units of a muscle, consist of protein molecules (actin and myosin). These proteins in the presence of calcium go through a chemical reaction that make them slide past each other (like fingers of both hands sliding into each other's spaces to lock hands), shortening the length and thickening up to produce what we call 'contraction', or more accurately 'shrinkage'. Actually, neither those proteins nor the muscle bulk contract in the true sense of the word. Muscles flex and extend, unlike solids which contract when cool and expand when heated. Muscle groups are classified as flexors when they move parts of the body together, and extensors when they move them apart. Thus the biceps of the arm is a flexor muscle because shortening it brings the hand closer to the shoulder and triceps is an extensor muscle as it does the opposite. Here flexion and extension are used to describe the movements. The two muscles (biceps and triceps), however, both 'contract' or shorten to be able to produce these movements. Thus 'contraction' is not the correct word to describe the genuine function of muscles and, as we will see later in the book, this word contradicts certain phenomena that take place in muscles. It is, however, only a technicality.

Muscles were studied electrically and under the electron microscope to determine their extraordinary functions. Nowadays, of course, there are more sophisticated methods of analysis and study. In the past, muscle 'contractions' were studied with the electrical impulses applied to them. Weights were placed to see if their length or their tone remained constant (isometric or isotonic contractions). The electron microscopic studies were used to study their structure (or morphology). Thus slow-, intermediate- and fast-twitching muscles were discovered. These muscles differ from each other structurally, as we have seen, in that they can contain different quantities of mitochondria, blood vessels and myoglobin. Their structural differences determine their endurance and their locations in the body depend on what work they are expected to perform. Thus spinal muscles are redder (as they have more blood and myoglobin) and they consist of slow-twitching muscles. Therefore they can contract for a long time without getting fatigued so easily. The muscles of the legs are paler in colour as they are expected to work fast and intensively. They get tired quite easily. That is because they have fewer mitochondria or less blood supply and depend on an anaerobic conversion of glucose that leads to lactic acid formation. All these discoveries were very exact and helped to understand why different muscles function differently.

The main problem is that the muscles were studied outside the human body *in vitro* (experimentally). What happens to the electrical circuit present in a living person is not exactly the same as in experimental situations. The studying of muscles *in vivo* (in a live person) is not only inhuman but quite difficult as it would be very painful. As it is, EMG (electromyogram) is used to study muscle function and, like bone-marrow biopsy, lumbar puncture etc, is a very painful investigation. In a living person the muscles receive more information than just the 'electrical impulse' from the nerve that makes them flex.

Muscle tone is a basic phenomenon seen in a living body. The flesh separated from the bone has no tone and so it is flaccid. Muscle tone not only creates the contours of muscles but also keeps them in the state of preparedness. Moreover, the tone keeps the body intact. As I mentioned earlier, stroke victims have frequent dislocation of the shoulder and hip joints. These ball and socket joints are kept in position not only by the ligaments but also by the tone of the muscles around them. Thus in a paralysed limb, the muscles are atonic and fail to keep the ball of the limb bone in the socket of the main bone. The sheer weight of the limb pulls it out of its natural position, thus causing the dislocation. This dislocation further impairs the function of the affected limb as it cannot move very well when the joint becomes dysfunctional.

Muscle Tone

Everybody has experienced the negative effects of muscles at some time or another. After a good afternoon nap one often feels listless with no energy to get up and walk. The body feels very heavy and lethargic. If one is exhausted, the muscles become very fatigued and lose most of their tone. Without muscle tone no physical activity is possible.

Loss of muscle tone not only increases the inertia but contributes extra heaviness to the body. As mentioned earlier, a sleeping child, a dead body or a paralysed person feels heavier than an active person. This happens for a variety of reasons and one is lack of muscle tone. In a stroke victim, where one half of the body is paralysed, the affected side feels heavier than the healthy one. The same blood flows through both the limbs and even though the affected side has weak or atrophied muscles with less volume, it feels heavier. Muscle tone is the only reason for this disparity in apparent weight, because the affected side does not have it.

Muscle tone is created by the subconscious part of the brain. Although these skeletal muscles are supposed to be controlled by a voluntary process of the

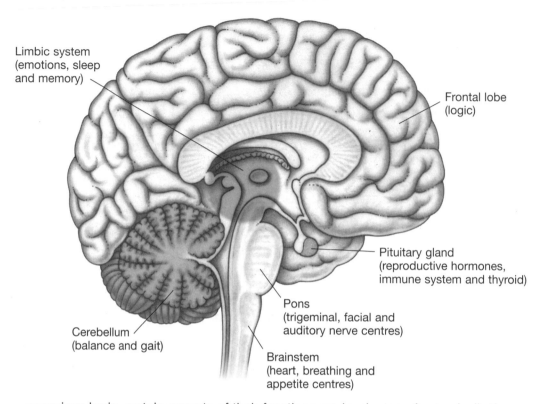

Limbic system
(emotions, sleep
and memory)

Frontal lobe
(logic)

Pituitary gland
(reproductive hormones,
immune system and thyroid)

Pons
(trigeminal, facial and
auditory nerve centres)

Cerebellum
(balance and gait)

Brainstem
(heart, breathing and
appetite centres)

conscious brain, certain aspects of their functions are involuntary. Anatomically the thalamus and cerebellum control gait, posture and muscle tone (see Figure above). These structures lie deep within the subconscious brain. In the thalamus there are nerve centres that control gait and muscle tone. When these centres are affected, due to lack of an essential chemical in them (domamine), the muscle tone and gait are affected and one becomes Parkinsonian. This is characterised by tremors, loss of facial expression and slow gait followed by sudden speeding up. These symptoms arise out of abnormalities of muscle tone. Excess tone leads to tremor and lack of it causes sluggishness.

Medical science has not been able to study the functions of the subconscious brain, though it has gone as far as mapping the brain to show where different control zones are located. As detailed studies would have to be done *in vivo*, the task is virtually impossible. (It's rather like trying to find out how a computer works by X-raying it to see where all the components are located, without having the faintest idea what goes on inside the chips.) Here again, logic is our best bet to prove that such phenomena must be happening. Muscle tone is controlled by the involuntary system, as the conscious brain would simply not be able to manage with such a mammoth task. Therefore, muscle tone is just there whether we experience or control it or not. Exercises do help to build it up, but the threshold level, that which is always there, is beyond our control under normal circumstances.

Finally, medical science has left the question of how we control muscle tone unanswered. It vaguely describes it as a basal state of 'contraction' of muscles at rest and the source of control was mapped in the brain.

What makes the human body stand erect?

This question has not been answered at all. Just like everything else, medical science attributed this force to the skeletal muscles of the spine as if it were held erect by guy ropes. This is the origin of all mistakes related to the problems of the spine. According to conventional medicine, the contraction of muscles in the spine keeps the vertebral column erect like a bamboo stick, which provides the scaffolding that holds the entire body weight. (In its defence I should add that bad posture can lead to spinal muscles interfering with the deep posture-maintaining muscles, resulting in a reduction in the effectiveness of the latter. Thus if tests are carried out on someone with bad posture it may well appear that the spinal muscles are contributing to the posture.)

The Spinal Discs

The vertebral column, they say, like a bamboo stick, has many joints on which the weight is supported. These joints are the discs, which get compressed due to injury or lack of muscle power or gain in weight. These compressed discs can press on nerve roots to cause pain and sometimes they damage the nerves to the extent that they cause neurological problems (pain, weakness in corresponding muscles, numbness, tingling etc). It is concluded that all back problems seem to stem from the discs and they are therefore the target of all back treatments. If the discs are not degenerate or they do not bulge then there is no backache or other problems related to the spine. Therefore, discs are scooped out, they are partially resected, the corresponding vertebrae are fused to make them immobile to avoid pressure on the disc and they are partially sucked out. These are the various surgical tactics used to treat disc-related problems.

Those who treat backache conservatively will start with anti-inflammatory drugs and prolonged total backrest (often for two weeks or more) so the inflammation is reduced, then use traction to 'decompress' the disc (often causing more agony). Manipulation is employed 'to bring the discs back into position' by adjusting the facet joints (those that link vertebrae together) with exercises to 'strengthen the back'. One may be advised to lose some weight to 'reduce the pressure on discs'. The exercises that are prescribed range from stretching to swimming and light weightlifting. These exercises 'tone up' the muscles and relieve the pain by holding the spine together.

The above completes the chain reaction.

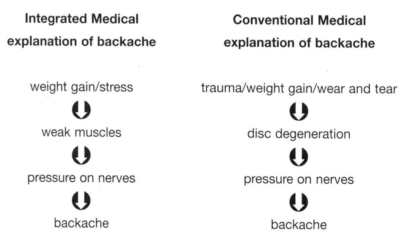

Integrated Medical	**Conventional Medical**
explanation of backache	**explanation of backache**
weight gain/stress	trauma/weight gain/wear and tear
⬇	⬇
weak muscles	disc degeneration
⬇	⬇
pressure on nerves	pressure on nerves
⬇	⬇
backache	backache

Treating the Pain Ignores the Cause

Thus a common problem like backache, which can potentially ruin people's lives, is managed by medicine in a mechanistic way. Discs cause the problem so they are removed to relieve the pain or treated. If tonsils cause recurrent problems they are treated with antibiotics or are removed. Teeth are conservatively treated or removed to relieve the pain. No mention is ever made of what causes these areas to degenerate or get inflamed in the first place. Since it is not exactly known what causes discs to be maintained in status quo or what force keeps the spine erect, the immediate culprit (the discs) is therefore attacked. Thus backache becomes chronic and in the majority of cases it remains as a potential health hazard. Once a backache, always a backache is the slogan. Some people get over it and keep it at bay with weight control and regular exercises. If they stop they know that it will come back and often with a vengeance, causing great personal discomfort. One is always aware of backache. There isn't a single person in the urban world who has never experienced backache, in some form or another. It is universal even though some people may not notice it when the pain is subthreshold. A person experiences pain when it crosses a certain barrier or threshold. Problems like disc compression may start long before the actual symptoms appear and the discomfort caused to the back in this phase remains unnoticed because it remains in the subthreshold zone.

Journey to Find the Cause of Back Pain

Now, returning to the main question, what keeps us erect, I have logically approached it and carried out personal observation for over 20 years. In 1982 when I returned to Delhi after my postgraduation in Moscow, armed with a medical degree, diplomas and certificates in acupuncture, fasting therapy, hypnotherapy, iridology, homoeopathy etc, I was faced with a difficult task of setting up an integrated medical practice, blending the knowledge I had acquired. By good fortune I was able to open a clinic.

In India there are many homoeopaths, Ayurvedic physicians and naturopaths, so at first I could not convince people to come to me. Acupuncture, however, was something new, so I projected myself as a specialist in this area, though I wanted to be an integrated medical physician practising elements of everything I knew.

By sheer coincidence people approached me for treatment of backache and arthritis, two common conditions that are treated with acupuncture. Thus I had no choice but to treat these conditions for work experience and financial support. In Moscow, I'd treated all sorts of conditions from bronchial asthma to migraine, but in New Delhi, before I became well-known in my field, I was known as 'the best back man'.

As a postgraduate student in Moscow, I had taken a brief course in massage under a well-known physiotherapist, Ms Miranova. She was tall, heavy and indeed very tough in her treatment. She did a very deep massage to stimulate the muscles of the body for various types of physical conditions. Under her expert hands patients would moan and groan but come out thoroughly invigorated and refreshed. At first I found the massage tough as my fingers and hands were more used to doing such delicate things as writing, acupuncture and pulse reading. Pressing the muscles, kneading and pummelling required different skills altogether. I had learnt her technique, however, thinking it might come in handy one day and so it did, in Delhi.

I would massage the back for a few minutes before inserting acupuncture needles to relieve backache. People would get tremendous relief from this combined effect. Some people, however, especially women, were very scared of needles as they would imagine the worst possible scenario of pain and agony. I then had no option but to restrict my therapy to massage only. The results were just as good and after many such experiences I realised that massage was a powerful method of treatment of backache in itself. I therefore switched over to massage and yogic exercises for treatment of back problems and related complications like sciatica. Soon the word got around and my appointment book filled up with back sufferers. When I opened an evening clinic in West Delhi, most of the patients that came to see me suffered from backache.

Over the past 20 years, I have treated thousands of backaches of different types and developed my own technique. My natural curiosity made me probe into this and find out why my method of treatment worked so well. By touching and feeling muscles and ligaments I was able to discover the various defects in them. My knowledge of applied anatomy (anatomy as applied to a human body) helped me to identify precisely the various structures like strains of muscles, ligaments, joints, tendons and their pathology (sprain, tear, inflammation, disalignment etc). It is this knowledge combined with a dedicated effort to seek the truth, that helped me to discover the clues to various types of back problems. One who searches finds, provided one is dedicated enough to persevere.

All this time I was making my own study of people's backs. I experimented with various aspects of my technique and drew my own conclusions. Thus I benefited immensely from these treatments and practice certainly makes one perfect. So I discovered the various causes of pain, spasms of muscles and scoliosis and found treatments for them.

This went on for almost 10 years before I formulated my hypothesis and proved it in my own mind with practice and logic. I discovered that medical science had lost its way in understanding and teaching backache, as some initial blunders on the understanding of functions of muscles had led to confusion on the subject. I also realised that it is sometimes not merely a physical problem but a complex psychological and emotional problem leading to a physical manifestation.

Years later in London my colleague, Miss Jiwan Brar, who specialised in therapeutic yoga after completing a course in physical therapy and sports injury management, helped me with an assessment of the various back conditions. Having been a PhD scholar at King's College in London in genetics, she was very methodical and scientifically orientated. I discussed my hypothesis of posture management and backache and she helped me to evaluate those ideas, with brilliant results. Time and again she tested chronic backache cases assessing the state of the weight-bearing and other involuntary muscle fibres. We treated many of these patients together. I did the massage/manipulative therapy, while she used specific yoga exercises, designed for backaches, to treat the most complicated cases that came to me. I had used simple yogic exercises in the past but Jiwan developed a series of highly effective therapeutic yoga exercises in line with my hypothesis and concept of the muscle functions. We worked together for years perfecting the technique which became known in the clinic as **THE ALI TECHNIQUE FOR BACKACHE**.

Chapter 4

Logical Analysis of Posture

Experiment 1

Lie on your back, put both hands on the abdominal muscles on either side your navel. Raise your head and try to sit up feeling the tension in the rectus abdominis (rectal muscles of the abdomen). You will notice the extreme tightness of these muscles as you slowly sit up. Notice what happens when you finally reach your destination and sit up erect. You are in for a bit of a surprise at this point. The taut muscles of the abdomen after completion of their involuntary movements suddenly become flaccid. Therefore, these abdominal muscles and the muscles on the inner lining (anterior spinal muscles) of the spine perform just one function: namely raising the body from horizontal to the vertical sit-up position and play very little role in maintaining the erect posture. Once the motion is complete their role finishes and some other groups of muscles seem to take over to make you sit erect.

Experiment 2

Sit on a chair and put your hands on both thighs, gently squeezing the quadriceps or thigh muscles. Get up slowly and notice the tightness or tension in these muscles as you go up. Just as you acquire the vertical position and release the control over these muscles, they will become instantaneously

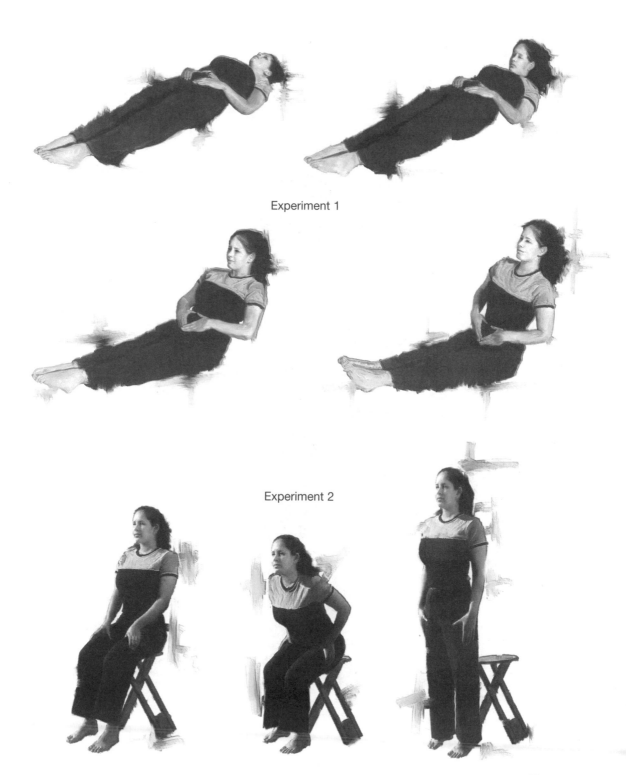

Experiment 1

Experiment 2

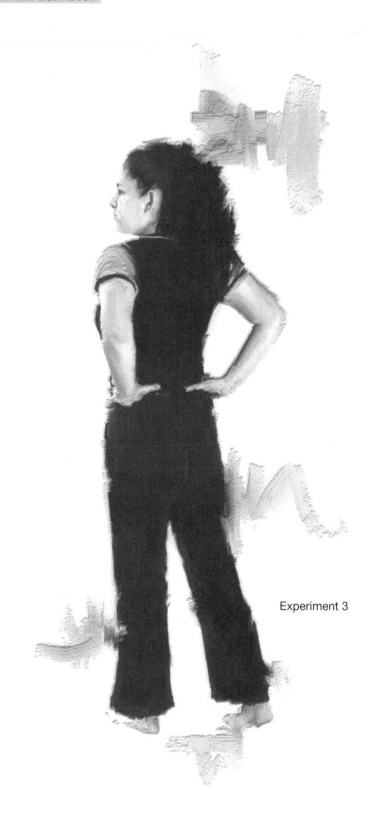

Experiment 3

flaccid. One might expect these muscles to be taut so as to support the body in the vertical position but that does not happen.

Experiment 3

Put both thumbs on either side of the lumbar spine on the low back muscles pressing into them. Then walk slowly and feel how one side or the other contracts as you lift one leg and put the other on the floor while walking. Stand still and march on the spot doing the same thing. An amazing phenomenon will be noticed. The side on which the leg is raised is more tight or taut than the other which bears the weight of the body. This is an irony, as putting all your weight on one side, as opposed to both sides, should tighten the lumbar muscle concerned. This does not happen and in fact the muscles are quite normal in their tension. There is hardly any noticeable increase in tension of spinal muscles on the side on which you stand.

Conclusions

These simple experiments prove logically that voluntary (those which 'contract' at will) skeletal muscles of the spine or the lower limbs play very little role in maintaining the erect posture. Yet the body stands upright so there must be other muscle fibres, which we cannot control at will, that keep it that way.

These muscle fibres get their information from the posture and balance centres in the subconscious brain. Impulses from these centres must be maintaining the equilibrium of posture as the burden of carrying out this function is too much to handle for the conscious mind. The latter is so specialised in its functions that it carries out the higher psychic, intellectual and voluntary activities only. Nature has not loaded it with the additional responsibilities of carrying out routine and mundane functions or activities like gait, posture, digestion, breathing etc. If that had happened the conscious brain would have had very little energy or capacity to make decisions. Nature thus separated the conscious and subconscious brain, providing separate circulatory systems and entrusting them with different functional roles.

Different Muscle Fibres

It seems that within the same muscle there are different types of muscle fibre carrying out different functions. This can be clearly seen in the third experiment with the marching on the spot. The tightness of muscles on the side where the leg has been lifted shows (a) that movement has been carried out and (b) that the weight of the limb has been borne by these muscles. The relatively relaxed state of the muscles in the opposite side shows that posture maintaining or indirect weight-bearing muscles carry out their functions without tightening. Thus inside one large muscle or muscle group there are different types of muscle fibres carrying out separate functions.

Medical science has not dealt with this aspect of the functionally different muscle fibres. It has gone as far as describing slow, intermediate and fast muscle fibres but not as far as classifying muscle fibres into the ones that shrink and the ones that don't. Clearly, there seem to be two or possibly more types of muscle fibres. Nobody has proved it but logically it seems to be true.

It seems that the muscle fibres that support posture do not need to tighten up into a hard 'knot' when 'contracting'. Even when extra weight is added on, they don't seem to tighten up at all. Weightlifters when lifting heavy weights experience tightness of the back muscles only when they lift the weight from the stand to the overhead position, but once they have achieved their final static position and the spine is erect, the back muscles return to normal tone and don't feel tight any more. One can try a similar experiment with a partner who puts the thumbs on the lumbar muscles to feel their tightness or softness during lifting of a heavy object from the ground to over the head.

Elongation of Muscles

From these simple experiments it becomes obvious that one type of muscle moves, lifts and carries weight by tightening up or shrinking (all shrinking muscle fibres flex or draw up into each other to form a hard mass of flesh). There seems to be another group of muscles that do the opposite, i.e. elongate and thin out. This latter group of muscles is the one that most definitely supports the posture. That is why such muscles do not tighten up into a hard mass. The process of elongation 'thins the bulk of the muscles' and this results in relative softening up of muscles. F. M. Alexander (who invented the Alexander Technique for posture control and incidentally was an actor, not a doctor) may have been the first to point out this elongation and the curious fact that a muscle is more powerful when it is lengthening than when it is shortening. Indeed, Professor F. P. Jones researching the Alexander Technique at Tufts University in Boston was able to show by X-ray that Alexander movements brought about lengthening of the sternocliedomastoid muscles in the neck, with a related increase in width of the discs between the neck vertebrae (Stevens 1987). Other research into the Alexander Technique established that muscles are more powerful when they expand than when they contract.

In the first experiment I described on page 38, as soon as the body attains the vertical position and stops, the posture-maintaining/supporting muscles switch into action instantaneously and the tight muscles of the abdomen or spine become soft or flaccid. There is a quick transfer of power, so quick that it is almost a smooth transition.

In the second experiment, as soon as the vertical position is achieved the quadriceps stop acting as muscles that help to move the body from a sitting position to an erect position and become muscles that maintain posture (vertical). Therefore, the quadriceps too have two distinct groups of muscles, one participating in walking, kicking, jumping etc while the other group elongates and supports the torso's weight. The first group causes tightening of quadriceps while the other doesn't.

In the third experiment, the side of the back that lifts the leg is tight while the other, that supports weight, is soft. Here both groups of muscles function in the opposite way. This is clear evidence of the two groups of muscles carrying out opposite types of function – one supports the weight of the leg and lifts, while the other elongates to maintain posture. What is interesting in this experiment is that while the one group of muscle fibres tightened to lift and support the weight of the leg, the other group elongated to maintain posture on the same side. That is why, even when standing on one leg, the muscles that seem to be carrying extra weight do not feel any different from when the person stands on both legs. This is what happens all the time and in most of our activities. During walking, lifting, jumping etc these muscles have to maintain the vertical position too. Thus posture-maintaining muscles function independently from those muscles that carry out movements or lift weight.

In the third experiment, it can clearly be seen that posture-maintaining muscles elongate and push the weight upwards towards the sky. That is why they do not tighten up, even though they participate in supporting substantial weight. A heavy object or weight has a gravitational force directed down the arms, spine, abdomen and legs and this force is counteracted by another force, which is distinctly anti-gravitational. Thus the muscles that support posture can also support weight through an upward thrust or anti-gravitational force. If there were no upward (anti-gravitational) force, a heavy weight would bend the joints of arms and legs like a concertina and crush the discs of the spine. The substantial weight that the weightlifter carries (often up to 500 lbs) could not be held up without an active force directed upwards. This force counteracts the gravitational force created by the combined weight of the body and the weights, and creates a perfect balance or equilibrium. This neutralisation of the downward (gravitational) force is so harmonised that joints of wrists, elbow, shoulders, back, hips, knees, ankles and feet do not bend. They are kept in perfect alignment in the vertical position. What incredible engineering ingenuity created by Nature! Suddenly joints which by nature are mobile or flexible become perfectly aligned even in the most crucial period when a heavy weight has been lifted.

There is, however, a limit to how much weight these posture/weight-bearing muscles can support. As seen with weightlifters, the winner is the one that supports maximum weight through his training and endurance. Those who fail are either unable to lift the weight off the stand or they drop the weights before straightening the arms above the head as they feel there could be a potential risk of damage to the body. At this precise moment the joints bend and 'give in' sending signals of impending danger of tearing muscles. The discs in the lumbar spine are also at tremendous risk as they may get compressed beyond what is normal and suffer damage. That is why people who lift heavy weights or suddenly put on a lot of weight suffer low backaches quite frequently.

The fact that the body creates an anti-gravitational force to support its own weight as well as the added one, indicates that posture-maintaining or weight-bearing muscle fibres actually elongate or extend upwards against gravity. This conclusion is based on logic as almost no experiment or study has been carried out other than simple observations that I have made over the years and the isolated case of Professor F. P. Jones quoted opposite. As mentioned earlier, the main problem has been the fact that these experiments need to be carried out *in vivo* in a conscious person. This makes it difficult and 'unethical'.

I do know of one invasive study done by Nachemson in Sweden, where pressure-sensitive needles were inserted into the discs of living persons, showing that the pressure on discs is higher when sitting than when standing. The pressure was least when the subject was lying down, not surprisingly, but was three times as great when lying on one side or standing erect, five times as great when sitting upright, nine times as great when standing and bending forward and ten times as great when sitting and leaning forward. It is therefore greatly to your discs' and your posture-maintaining muscles' advantage to stand and sit upright, rather than bring the leaning muscles into play like guy ropes pressing down on a tent pole.

Role of muscle up-thrust

Pending scientific investigation and proof that these upward-stretching muscles are solely responsible for the human body's vertical posture and that these muscles not only bear the weight of the body but also relieve pressures on the joints and discs of the spine and major joints of the legs (like your palm muscles did to the marbles), we will have to accept these facts on the basis of logical conclusions. Science has in general failed to observe and study these phenomena over the decades. That is why backache and osteoarthritis ('wear and tear' of joints) of the major joints of the legs (hip, knees and ankles) are common and unresolved problems of medicine. It is common sense that any pressure taken off the joints of the leg and discs and joints of the spine would prevent them from injury, degeneration and inflammation. The less the load or pressure, the less the 'wear and tear'.

The fact that I concluded over years of study of muscles, backache and joint problems, that the body's own anti-gravitational force prevents these injuries taking place, is potentially a major contribution to medical science. As we will see later, by building up this upward thrust or the anti-gravitational force, not only can we eliminate pain, inflammation, degeneration of discs and joints but also prevent backache and osteoarthritis in the legs that are caused by 'wear and tear'. It must, however, be remembered that there are other causes of osteoarthritis ranging from nutritional factors to trauma.

The upward thrust or anti-gravitational force created by muscles is subconsciously controlled. That is why during the various experiments mentioned earlier in this chapter, one sees a sudden transition from what can be controlled and regulated to something beyond the conscious brain. The change is so subtle that the moment of transfer is quite amazing. As mentioned earlier, this function is controlled by specific gait and posture centres in the mid-brain and cerebellum, which are subcortical or of the subconscious brain.

Voluntary/involuntary control

There are muscles in the body that are both voluntarily and involuntarily controlled. Here are some examples:

1

The diaphragm can be made to 'contract' voluntarily by the conscious brain, although most of the time it moves involuntarily. That is why we are not normally aware of our breathing, it is just an automatic process. Those who practise 'pranayama' or yogic breathing voluntarily guide the diaphragm to breathe correctly. It is expected that normally a person should breathe like a child, who blows the belly out while breathing in and takes the belly in while exhaling. That is the correct way of breathing. Most people, unconsciously, do the reverse. They take the abdomen in while inhaling and blow it out when exhaling. With regular practice and training one can switch over to the correct breathing pattern which then becomes automatic or subconsciously controlled.

2

The anal sphincter is involuntarily controlled. Just before defecation the sphincter opens on its own and the stool masses are pushed out. However, with the help of the muscles on the pelvic floor, the anal stricture can be achieved. The anal muscles can be made to constrict and close the passageway. In fact, this voluntarily exercise (pelvic floor exercise) is recommended to people with prostate, bladder and haemorrhoids to improve these conditions. This exercise also helps pelvic flow. Those who have uncontrolled bowel movements and are prone to accidents, especially with the mucus or diarrhoea-type of Irritable Bowel Syndrome, can also be helped with these involuntary exercises.

3

When a child learns to write A, B, C, D etc. he is taught to move the fingers in a particular way to write these letters. Later on the child begins to write sentences and is still using the conscious brain to carry out this voluntary activity. After a few years of training, the writing skill is developed and it becomes automatic. The thoughts are transferred into written words almost unconsciously. This skill is developed. All skills are intuitive by nature and are borderline with the subconscious brain. Similar things happen with typing when the fingers automatically 'know' where the letters are on the keyboard. Driving is a skill and the footwork on the brake and accelerator become automatically controlled. Most people drive with minimum concentration and active use of the conscious brain. They talk on the mobile phone, or to their companions, listen to music etc and drive subconsciously. The visual response and judgement of speed or distance between cars is almost automatic. It is scary to think that driving skill is mostly controlled on the fringe of the subconscious brain.

4

Speech when taught is voluntarily controlled. The child or a student learning a new language learns to pronounce words and sentences using the lips, tongue, teeth, etc. After a while the whole process becomes automatic. The words are formed in the conscious brain but are executed by the subconscious brain. The movement of the speech apparatus (breath, vocal cords, tongue, lips etc) is subconsciously controlled. This is why most people who learn a second language speak with an 'accent'. They have failed to retrain their brain to form new sounds like a native.

5

Gait is also subconsciously controlled. If the conscious brain were to control and coordinate all the muscles involved in gait and balance, there would be frequent mistakes resulting in falls and injuries. This does not happen as Nature has entrusted the most advanced and precise part of the brain, the subconscious, to deal with it. The conscious mind is all too vulnerable to external influences and too engrossed with the thinking process to be able to control delicate and precise movements.

Control of posture

Similarly posture is maintained by the subconscious brain. Again it shows the incredible ingenuity of Nature. Imagine the planning, the power and the skill that went into such a unique system of precise balance and posture control. A thousand computers could not mimic this effect. The body stands erect as a result of synchronised action by billions of individual muscle fibres controlled by an equal number of nerve impulses. The result is perfect balance and erect posture. Generally speaking there are several individual forces that act simultaneously to achieve the following:

a

To create an anti-gravitational force equal to the weight of the body plus the force required to keep the spine erect so that the delicate discs and joint surfaces are not traumatised by the weight of the body (the joints of the lower limbs are taken into consideration besides the spinal joints).

b

To prevent the body from falling over by creating opposite forces within the body that act from all directions to counteract gravitational forces that might want to topple the body. This is so obvious and can be felt clearly when standing on one leg or walking with eyes shut. One can then feel the tightening and loosening of various muscles in the spine and legs that coordinate so that the body does not fall.

c

To keep the head, spine, legs and feet aligned so that the various discs and joints are maintained in a harmonious and comfortable position. The idea is to minimise the trauma to them while they carry out their normal functions. While walking, sitting and playing sports, the body acquires all sorts of different positions and postures with the help of muscles and joints. The muscles of the body, particularly the ones controlled by the subconscious brain, work continuously to keep up with what the conscious brain wants by facilitating such postures or positions as well as preventing trauma to the various discs, joints and other parts of the body.

d

To support the abdominal organs. Most of the organs are in front of the spine (heart, liver, intestines, etc). Therefore there is a tendency to fall flat on one's face. Spinal muscles coordinate and create a 'pulley force' that brings the body to a balanced erect position.

All these forces act in perfect coordination with each other and the subconscious brain is in full charge of the situation. However, the functions of posture can also be consciously guided, like breathing muscles (diaphragm, intercostal muscles) which, although involuntary in most part, are also controllable. As will be discussed later, my technique for backache, the Alexander technique, Pilates and the Feldenkrais Method take full account of this fact. Posture can therefore be maintained and controlled. Nature has therefore given us dual control over these muscles so that when necessary the conscious brain has a say in the body's matters. Like everything else, it is an acquired skill and one has to make an effort to work towards a better posture. Writing, driving, correct pronunciation of words etc are all acquired skills. Posture too comes under this category and therefore is not fully automatic. It can be controlled at will. This is again another marvel of Nature.

Importance of posture

The muscles that support posture, I maintain, elongate or stretch against gravity to do so. Scientifically speaking this statement will bring the wrath of the medical community on me and I will be declared an eccentric instantly. I have worked a long time on backs and given posture extensive thought before daring to put it on paper.

It should not, however, come as any surprise. This has been practised for thousands of years by the military. Those of us who have done National Service remember the bark of the sergeant major. 'Stand up straight – head-up – shoulders back – chin in ...' All these tend to transfer the responsibility for posture from the fast-twitching superficial muscles to the long endurance slow-twitching deep postural muscles. No soldier who stooped could survive a route march. Indeed I am certain that survivors of the infamous 'death marches' of the Second World War were those who, despite the vicious whippings across the back, tending to make them bend over in pain, forced themselves upright, transferring their posture to the well-protected long endurance muscles, taking the strain off the injured superficial muscles, which were then given a chance to heal.

A soldier's chores, on the other hand, such as mending, scrubbing, digging and so on, are known as 'fatigues', involving as they do the fast-twitching muscles which much more quickly become tired or fatigued. Caesar's generals instinctively knew all this.

The point is, however, no one can at this time prove that my hypothesis is wrong. Indeed, logic and common sense prove it at once to be correct without scientific data. A child or a person who is slouching can be told to 'sit up straight' and you can see the changes in the spine. It pulls itself together and all the muscles of the back, abdomen and the sides coordinate to create an upward thrust. The result is an erect spine. If helped, the spine can really be stretched upward by several inches. While this happens the participating muscles thin out and feel less taut. Thus the elongation of muscles does not produce any tightness like those voluntary muscles that carry, lift and move the body and its parts. This explains why some muscles tighten when moving and are relaxed in the static position, as demonstrated in my experiments on movement and posture.

You can observe the same effect in Nature. Anyone who has been in close quarters to a cat when it leaps into a tree will have noticed that, as it leaves the ground, its length is momentarily greater than in any other posture it adopts.

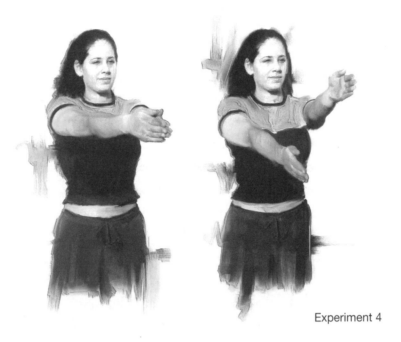

Experiment 4

Experiment 4

You can, however, do it yourself. Here is an experiment that may convince you that some muscle fibres can extend or elongate. On the inner surface of the hand, across the wrist just below the palm you will find two lines. Join these lines of both hands together and bring the palms of your hands together as in prayer. You'll see that the sizes of the fingers (when pressed together) of both hands are normally the same. Both palms of your hands and fingers are normally of the same dimension. Now raise one arm horizontally, take a deep breath in and breathe out slowly, imagining that your fingers are stretching out away from the palms. Imagine that some unknown force is pulling your fingers. Stretch them like this for a few times, reaching out for some mark on the wall. Then join the palms together starting with the lines below the palms and ending with the fingertips. You will notice that the fingers that were 'instructed' to stretch are longer than those on the other hand. This may surprise you as it is difficult to imagine that fingers can elongate at will. It does show, however, that muscles can stretch away from the body if the right instructions are given to them from the conscious brain.

Experiment 5

Here is another experiment to prove that even though posture-controlling muscles are controlled by the subconscious brain, the conscious part also plays a role. Stand in the 'attention' position as a soldier does and remain still. You can easily do that. Now, focus on the two heels and imagine that they are taking the entire weight of the body. Breathe in and out a few times and continue to focus on the heels and experience the weightlessness through the body. As soon as you feel this sensation you'll notice that your body will sway forward or backward as if you are losing balance. Corresponding muscles come into force to prevent this from happening. This experiment shows that the moment the conscious brain focuses on one part of the body, the posture-controlling forces that act right through the body lose their direction and as a result of that the state of equilibrium is lost. In the 'attention' position the body collects itself to maintain the most perfect posture but once that 'focus' is lost, everything seems to go berserk.

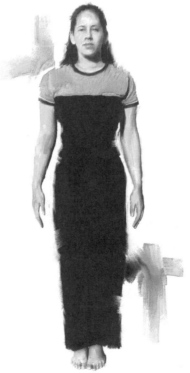

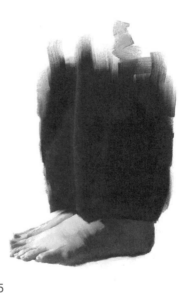

Experiment 5

Duality of Control

Therefore, the subconscious brain as well as the conscious brain plays a major role in maintaining posture and an erect position. In an unconscious state or in sleep the body will collapse. A person sleeping in a train cannot keep the head up and it sways in all possible directions in jerks. Similarly during a fainting attack the body collapses even though the subconscious brain functions quite well. A person who has fainted has normal breathing and pulse rate even though the consciousness is not there.

The ultimate example of elongating muscle fibres occurs during transcendental meditation (TM). All meditation creates a link between the conscious and subconscious mind, but TM has a physical manifestation. Its exponents adopt a sitting posture in such perfect balance that even the posture-maintaining muscles are not needed. There comes a point where the subconscious brain suddenly becomes aware that their support is missing and these muscles abruptly extend in synchronism, resulting in the sudden elongation of the spine by a matter of inches, like the marbles suddenly being squeezed. The jerk is so powerful that it lifts the body off the floor in a small leap. Some people refer to this as 'levitation'. It is, however, neither magic nor supernatural. It happens, it is well documented and easily explainable. I defy anyone, however, to explain it in a world in which muscles only contract.

So much for elongating muscles. I am sure there will still be sceptics who will argue that I have no scientific proof and therefore I must be wrong. This selective argument is often used by people who simply do not want to believe something, carefully glossing over those things they have to believe in but can't explain (such people probably wouldn't 'believe in' acupuncture or most of the functions of the brain). To those I say, all right don't believe it. Maybe there is some other explanation, that nobody has thought of yet, for the anti-gravitational force. Let us not argue about it. The fact is, and this is unarguable, that the posture-maintaining muscles and general muscle tone do create an anti-gravitational force that counteracts or neutralises part of the body's actual weight. In my concept of backache, this anti-gravitational force, created by posture-maintaining muscles and general muscle tone, plays a very important role. It is almost like the vital force of the back. The greater the force the less the pressure on the spine's joints and discs and on the joints of the leg.

Protection of the Spine

The fascinating thing about this force is, as I discovered over the years, that it actually determines the wear and tear of all the relevant structures as mentioned above. Thus if a disc degenerates and bulges or ruptures, it is most likely that it does so because of weakness of this vital anti-gravitational force. For the spinal discs and joints, nothing matters more than this force because the lack of it puts strain on them and the abundance of it relieves them from tension, creating flexibility and well-being.

Another fascinating aspect is that this anti-gravitational vital force can be increased through specific massages (passive treatment) and yogic exercises (active treatment). These treatments form an integral part of the Ali Technique for Backache. Most people who do spinal or general exercises, increase the general tone of muscles which form a minor part of the anti-gravitational force, indeed might actually increase it like guy ropes. Increase in posture-controlling muscle tone, however, relieves pain and removes some pressure from the affected or damaged discs, giving much needed relief in backache.

This force is weakened by a series of factors ranging from bad posture to fatigue to excess body weight with sluggish muscles. The reduction of this force leads to increased pressure on the spinal joints and discs, which in turn lead to inflammation of their surfaces causing pain and discomfort.

The anti-gravitational force created by posture-controlling muscles and general muscle tone is the most important factor for back health. Trauma, nutritional deficiencies, birth defects (like spina bifida), osteoarthritis, polymyalgia rheumatica etc appear in a relatively rare number of cases. Scientific medicine claims that the majority of backache cases originate from the discs and joints of the spine. Muscular and ligament sprains or inflammation form the second largest group of backache. If the anti-gravitational force in the living body is what determines the state of delicate spinal structures like joints, discs etc, the lack of it leading to backache and other related problems, then why haven't we looked at this over the centuries? Why did medicine go in the direction of treating symptoms only (pain, inflammation, nerve damage, scoliosis etc)? A branch called 'orthopaedics' (which someone once suggested to me translated as 'bone setting') was created, aimed at treating bones, joints and related hard tissues, which actually have hardly any primary role to play in the genesis of back-related problems. The bones and nerves are the final sufferers or victims of the weakening of another system, namely the muscular system, part of which, in a conscious state, produces an upward thrust that maintains the erect posture. This part of the muscular system is less voluntary and more involuntary, like the diaphragm muscles. Therefore, exercising it requires special skills as these muscles are under dual control, unlike skeletal muscles which are controlled entirely by the conscious brain.

Exercise

If skeletal or voluntary muscles that participate in lifting, carrying and movement, do not participate in maintaining erect posture, why then exercise them so vigorously to treat and prevent backache and back-related problems? So much money and hype have gone into the fitness industry from the latest gadgets to muscle-building supplements and yet, other than to create muscle tone and a general well-being through improved circulation and such vigorous exercises have little effect in curing and preventing backache. Sports persons, fitness instructors and numerous exercise enthusiasts suffer from the most excruciating backache ever. My honest feeling on the subject is that the fitter you are, the more severe the back problems are when you get them.

Back to Genesis

We have to change our attitude towards backache, by understanding the underlying forces and structures that cause it. Only then can we confidently go to the roots and eradicate the problem on a long-term basis and carry out preventive measures throughout our lives. That is the only way forward to solve a potentially debilitating and mostly chronic, not to mention very costly problem.

Chapter **5**

Anatomy and Physiology of the Backbone

Bone first appeared in the evolutionary chain more than 500 million years ago in primitive fish and became very common in many different groups of animals within about 100 million years. This was bone that provided mineral reserves, and protected these animals from predators by providing protective armour plating. The internal skeleton of these fish was composed of cartilage. During evolution this cartilage (soft bones) was replaced by bones.

Axial Skeleton

The human skeletal system is classified into the axial and appendicular divisions. The axial skeleton consists of bones of the skull, the vertebral column, the ribs and the sternum (breastbone). It is called axial because it forms the axis around which the main torso of the body is built. There are 80 bones in the axial skeleton and together they form roughly 40 per cent of all bones in the body.

The function of the axial skeleton is to create a framework that supports and protects the various internal organs (brain, heart, lungs etc) and provides extensive surface area for attachment of muscles that:

1

support the head

2

adjust the body's posture and position of the head, neck and trunk

3

move the spine

4

perform respiratory movement

5

stabilise or position structures of the appendicular skeleton (hip bone, bones of arms and legs, collarbone etc).

The joints of the axial skeleton are bound together by very powerful ligaments. This heavy reinforcement permits only limited movements of the axial skeleton. This is essential because a flexible central axis would not be able to keep the body's posture erect nor to support the weight of the various internal organs. The axial skeleton has to be strong and rigid or else it would be useless. Its strength lies in its inflexibility. The fact that bones are as strong as reinforced concrete and yet so light makes the axial skeleton function very effectively – it is light but extremely strong.

The main component of the axial skeleton is the vertebral column or the back-bone, as we commonly call it. This is the main support system for the torso and the head. Without this the body would never be able to stand erect and support its weight. It has, therefore, to be as strong as steel and yet be flexible when necessary. So it is another piece of brilliant engineering work by Nature or the Creator. It is there-fore important to understand the functions of the spinal column first, and the struc-tures that have developed to facilitate or carry out these functions. What are they?

Evolution

Let's start with a brief note on the evolution of the backbone, not in the very beginning, but at the level of the primates. When primates walked on all fours the spine was horizontal (as in dogs, horses, monkeys etc). The spine supported the weight of the various internal organs while the forelegs supported much of the weight of the body. The weight of the internal organs and the actual weight of the spine were supported by the back muscles.

Now this is important. Animals struck with a tranquillising dart collapse within minutes as the muscles of the legs and the spine collapse. Although the spine consists of tightly bound vertebrae, which give it great strength, on its own, without the muscles, it is not able to support internal organs (lungs, heart, liver, intestines, etc). Thus the spinal muscles attached to the various parts of the vertebral column of primates had to create a horizontal force that would keep the spine in that position. These muscles acted like steel wires or ropes and just as the weight of the washing is supported by a clothes line, so the weight of the visceral organs is supported by spinal muscles.

Let us look at some of the functions of the spine in general and see how the structure of the spine caters to these functions.

Human beings walk erect (since Homo Erectus in the evolutionary chain) and, therefore, the vertebrae of the spine become larger in the lower part to facilitate that. Just like the Eiffel Tower or a bamboo stem, which is thin at the top and becomes progressively thicker towards the base, the spinal vertebrae too become increasingly larger at the base of the spine so that the extra weight can be carried.

Discs

There are discs in the spinal column, in between the vertebrae. These discs, being filled with a gelatinous substance, provide a certain amount of cushioning and give mobility to the spine. If the discs were 'rock-solid' like bone, there would be no flexibility of the spine and bending forward or backward, rotational and natural movements would be impossible. Young bamboo shoots are extremely flexible but when the joints (discs) in them fuse as they mature, the flexibility is greatly reduced. There is an ailment of the backbone, ankylosing spondylitis (an autoimmune disease) where the spine joins up as a whole due to the calcification of the ligaments that bind the vertebrae together. The discs too solidify and thus appear like bamboo joints in an X-ray of the spine. This fusion leads to complete loss of flexibility of the back.

The discs in the human spine are very well developed while other animals do not have such a well-defined structure as they do not walk erect. The discs cushion the weight of the body, like shock absorbers. In a horizontal spine such a structure (discs) would be a hindrance to the spine as it would be difficult to maintain the rigidity to support the weight of the visceral organs.

The sizes of the discs vary in different parts of the spine. In the cervical (neck) area they are thinner and smaller and they become progressively larger and more developed down towards the lumbar spine. Their constituency becomes thicker and more fibrous tissue is found in the sheath that contains the disc fluid to form the 'disc'. So much so that the last intervertebral space between the last lumbar and first sacral vertebra is filled up with a very thick disc fluid, which generally calcifies by middle age and the two vertebrae almost fuse. This can happen prematurely as a resulting of the increase in wear and tear in today's tough world of stress and hyper-activity. This last disc takes the full weight of the trunk, head, arms and the various internal organs. It is the most vulnerable disc in the entire spine and maximum injury and resulting problems (pain, discomfort) take place at this level.

The last part of the vertebral column, the sacrum, is fused solid and the tail bones have shrunk to a symbolic representation owing to their obvious lack of use. The sacrum's units (vertebrae) have fused because its main function now is to provide a large joint surface or area for the hip bone so that it is able to support the bulk of the body weight. A smaller pair of joints, as in the rest of the vertebrae, would be too fragile and too small to carry out such a mammoth task of supporting the body weight. By fusing together and broadening, the sacrum provides a large surface area to which the joints as well as numerous spinal muscles attach themselves. This joint between the sacrum and the hip bone (ilium) is called the sacroiliac joint. It repre-sents the point where the spine and the hip meet. This joint has to be strong and inflexible as it is inconceivable to think how a mobile structure could remain steady while supporting such weight. It is therefore fused but with some mobility still remaining. That is why the sacroiliac joint (SIJ) often gets mildly disaligned and produces discomfort. As this joint has some soft tissues that are surrounded by thick sheaths of ligaments, they are prone to inflammation (a bone is solid and does not have blood vessels on the surface to produce inflammation). Painful sacroiliac joints are the commonest cause of lumbago and low backache. These joints are subjected to a lot of strain.

Lateral Projections

Finally, the vertebrae have many bony projections to which muscles and ligaments are attached. The long projections in the back of the vertebrae (one of them, the seventh cervical vertebra's posterior projection, sticks out in the upper back and is the one that creates the 'Dowager's hump') are useful for attachment of powerful ligaments which literally fix the vertebral column.

There are other lateral projections on either side of the vertebrae, called the transverse processes. These provide ample surface area for the attachment of the various spinal muscles (see Figure below). These transverse processes are interconnected with each other by powerful ligaments and muscles. The transverse processes in the thoracic region provide articulation or joint surfaces to which the ribs are attached.

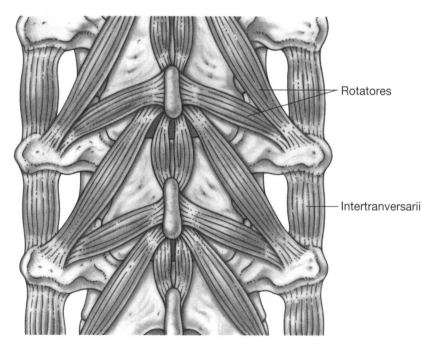

Rotatores

Intertranversarii

Intervertebral muscles

Spinal curves

1 Cervical

2 Thoracic

3 Lumber

4 Sacral

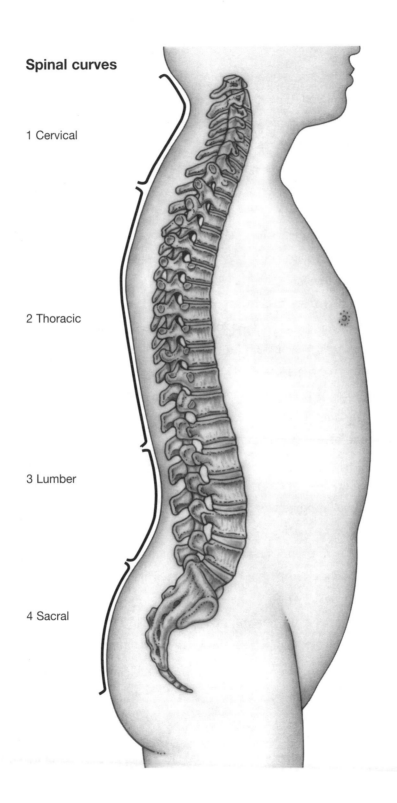

Curvature

Let us now look at the vertebral column as a whole. It consists of 7 cervical vertebrae, 12 thoracic vertebrae, 5 lumbar vertebrae and 5 sacral vertebrae, which fuse completely between 25 to 30 years of age. The total length of the vertebral column of an adult averages 28 inches.

The vertebrae do not form a straight and rigid structure. If you look at the spine from the side (see Figure on page 61) you will see that it has several curves, namely (1) the cervical curve, (2) the thoracic curve, (3) the lumbar curve and (4) the sacral curve.

The thoracic and sacral curves are called primary curves as they appear by the end of foetal development and are present in the newborn. They are also called 'accommodation curves' as they accommodate the thoracic organs (lungs, heart and other related structures) and abdominal and pelvic organs (large intestines, small intestines, uterus, kidney, bladder, rectum etc). These organs are voluminous and they need space, so the spine in the thoracic and sacral regions curves out (convex) to accommodate these organs. In the case of the sacrum, the weight of the abdominal organs tends to push them downwards into the pelvic region where they need ample space to be accommodated.

As the child learns to raise its head or stand erect, the secondary curves or compensation curves appear to compensate for the weight put on the spine. Thus the cervical curve appears when the child raises its head and tries to hold the head up. The weight of the relatively heavy head creates this curve, by caving in (concave). The lumbar curve appears when the weight of the trunk or upper part of the body is required to be supported by the lumbar spine. This happens as the child learns to stand erect and walk. At age ten all four curves of the spine appear.

Several abnormal curves may appear during childhood and adolescence. During this developmental stage, nutritional problems, abnormal weight gain, stress, posture problems, trauma etc may cause one or other of the abnormal curves. The main ones are:

Kyphosis (Ki-fo-sis)

which is an exaggerated thoracic curvature ('hunchback' type of curve).

Lordosis

which is an exaggerated lumbar curvature (people with huge bellies may have this)

Scoliosis

which is an abnormal lateral curvature. This can be noticed not from the sides but from the back. Instead of the spine being more or less straight, it produces curves to the sides. There are several reasons for this type of abnormal lateral curvature. Psychological problems in childhood or adolescence are the most common. In a later chapter, I will discuss this problem in detail.

When one stands erect, one's weight is transmitted through the spine on to the hip and ultimately to the lower limbs. Yet most of the weight of the body is in front of the spine (all the internal organs – heart, lungs, liver, intestines, uterus etc are in front of the spine). The various curves in the spine pull the various organs back to bring that weight in line with the body's axis. Thus these curves help to support the weight of the various organs as well as keep this weight balanced in the vertical position. A flexible plastic rod when pressed down on the floor or ground will develop curves to maintain the weight. These curves act like springs to accommodate the weight of the body. If one puts on a lot of weight and the spinal muscles are weak then these curves may be accentuated, causing problems. The discs are not the only shock absorbers. In fact the curvatures provide an element of shock absorption as well.

Consider yourself carrying a heavy weight in your hands. The natural reaction would be for you to increase or exaggerate the lumbar curvature to be able to evenly balance the weight, through the compensatory change in curve. If the weight is heavy, you will feel constrained in your lower back. Similar things happen in late pregnancy. Due to the increase in weight in the abdomen the lumbar curve increases and women get a continuous low backache. If they do not prepare themselves with exercises, the condition becomes very uncomfortable. People who have put on a lot of weight face similar problems.

In the case of women carrying weight (pitcher, fodder etc) on their heads in certain countries like Africa and India, the weight is distributed along the axis of the spine and weight-bearing muscles create the upward thrust, neutralising the load. This does not result in any increase in the spinal curves. Similarly men with powerful spinal muscles do not have exaggerated lumbar curves when they put on weight as the excess weight is well compensated for.

Common Structure of Vertebrae

If one looks at the main individual vertebrae, i.e. cervical, thoracic and lumbar, then they have the following common structures and characteristics:

 a

they have an arch with a spine and this arch forms a tunnel through which the spinal cord passes. The spinal cord, being a very delicate structure carrying nerve cables, needs the same protection that the skull offers the brain.

b

the arches rest on flat and round structures called the 'bodies' of the vertebrae. These are the platforms on which the arches rest but their main function is that they articulate with other bodies of vertebrae (above and below this particular one) by means of the discs. Thus the bodies of the vertebrae are interconnected by discs (i.e. two connect with each vertebra – one above and one below). These bodies provide the ligaments, the surface area and the cushions that are necessary for the tough but gelatinous discs to be housed. Discs, therefore, are sandwiched between the bodies of the vertebrae. The body of a vertebra has joints (facet joints) by means of which it can be linked to the vertebrae above and below. Finally, the bodies of the vertebrae have lateral projections (transverse processes) to which ribs and powerful back muscles are attached.

Cervical Vertebrae

The cervical spine has flat vertebrae which are supported by smaller ligaments and have numerous muscles attached to them. These muscles help the spine to move in different planes. The top two vertebrae of the neck (C1 and C2) are different from all other vertebrae of the spine. The second one, called the axis, has a finger-like projection around which the first one rotates. This gives the head freedom to rotate sideways, without actually forcing the entire neck to do so. The first one (C1) has a pair of large joint surfaces upon which the skull rests like a bowl of soup (see Figure on page 159). This first vertebra is named after the Greek Titan, Atlas, who supported the heavens (head) above the world (body).

Because of the smaller and flatter vertebrae and numerous weak muscles and ligaments, the cervical spine is not as toughly bound together as the thoracic and lumbar vertebrae. This part of the spine is more prone to injuries, sprains and dislocation of joints. Rotational injuries usually take place in the first three vertebrae, as they are free to move in clockwise and anti-clockwise directions. Injuries from the side can dislocate any joint and cause disalignment of the cervical spine.

The cervical spine has another distinct feature. Each of the seven vertebrae has a hole in the lateral projections. These holes form a canal of bones interconnected with tough ligaments in the spaces between these lateral projections (see Figure on page 164). This canal is called the vertebral canal and contains on each side the most vital arteries and veins of the entire body – the vertebral arteries and veins. As I will discuss later, these blood vessels, especially the arteries that take blood to the subconscious brain, are very important as they literally control our entire existence. These are the only blood vessels in the body to be provided such protection. Furthermore, the protection has to be maintained in a highly flexible and mobile environment. This strength, however, can also be a weakness. Though it protects the arteries from direct damage, a fault in the protection, such as dislocation of a cervical vertebra, can restrict the channel and hence the supply of blood to the subconscious brain. This accounts for many symptoms, as we will see later, that apparently have nothing to do with the spine.

Role of Vertebrae

We therefore see that the vertebrae or the vertebral columns are designed by Nature to meet the demands of the functions of the spine. Each of their structures carry out a certain function. If we understand the role that the vertebral column or an individual vertebra carries out, we can easily understand their structure(s). Everything is there for a purpose. For example, the discs cushion the vertebrae, acting as 'springs' or 'shock absorbers'; the bony canals protect the spinal cord and the vertebral arteries;

the various projections provide the surface areas for the muscle and ligament attachments and so on.

Disc Conditions

As mentioned earlier, the majority of backache in the lumbar region stems from disc degeneration or abnormalities (rupture and bulge of discs). Therefore, it is important to know exactly what the discs consist of and why they cause problems when things are not right.

Intervertebral discs or discs located between the vertebrae (from third cervical to the sacrum) have tough outer layers of fibrocartilage, known as 'annulus fibrosis'. This is a very tough sheath whose collagen fibres are attached to the bodies of the vertebrae above and below. These attached fibres give the discs stability and strength, which allows the bulk of the disc some sort of stability. The disc is thus fixed to the bodies of the vertebrae.

The disc can be compared to a round hot-water bottle. The rubber part is the fibrous 'annulus fibrosis' and the water inside the bottle is represented by a soft, elastic and gelatinous core known as 'nucleus pulposis' (pulp-like nucleus or core). The nucleus pulposis gives the disc resiliency and enables it to act as a shock absorber. About 75 per cent of the core is water and the rest is scattered reticular and elastic fibres. This makes the pulp or core of the disc gelatinous and facilitates its function as a shock absorber.

Movement of the vertebral column compresses the nucleus pulposis and displaces it in the opposite direction, which permits smooth gliding movements of each vertebra while still maintaining their alignment. The springs of a car allow movement of the axle with respect to the chassis, like muscles, while the shock absorbers prevent the sharp thumps of the road from overstretching the springs, like discs. The vertebrae can also move sideways, laterally or rotate, but they remain attached to the discs, which take up the shocks.

The axis of rotation of vertebrae is towards the front of each vertebra, not in the centre. They do not rotate about the disc, so the disc is always sliding a little. Slipping is part of the natural action of the disc. The expression 'slipped disc' is therefore misleading. Between the lower vertebrae the disc is attached to the bone above and below. Imagine a hot-water bottle again filled with fluid, which you hold between your hands, one above the other below. As you rotate your arms about the elbows in opposite directions, one flat side of the bottle moves with respect to the other. Thus it is the muscles that provide support during rotation or tilting, like car springs, while the disc is the shock absorber or cushion. It is not part of the rotation, in fact it wobbles like the hot-water bottle. Similarly the cartilage in the knee, the meniscus, is just a shock absorber. It doesn't play any role in the rotation. All these are shock absorbers. Discs, however, are soft while the cartilage in the knee is tough.

The discs make a significant contribution to the height of a person. On an average, they account for one quarter of the length of the vertebral column. Thus, as we grow older and there is a loss of moisture in these discs, this causes the spine to shrink. This explains the loss in height in elderly people. With age the discs lose their ability to cushion or absorb shock as they become degenerated. This increases the risk of rupture or what people call 'slipped disc', though it is actually caused by the disc losing the capacity to slip.

Besides the intervertebral discs there are two pairs of articulations (facet joints) between the upper and lower vertebrae. These are gliding joints between adjacent vertebrae and they permit small movements associated with flexion (bending forward) and rotation (turning sideways) in the vertebral column. These movements have to be restricted as there are very sensitive structures, such as nerves emerging out of the spinal cord, which may otherwise be damaged. Movements in these joints are restricted by numerous ligaments, tendons and smaller muscles that firmly bind the vertebrae together. The vertebral column is designed to maintain a steady upward position and its movement is very limited. Sudden movements as in a fall or injury can tear the ligaments and muscles that bind these vertebrae. Stress and strain can also weaken these soft tissues. When that happens the chances of these facet joints dislocating is very high. Wrong movements or sudden jerks can dislocate these joints. This results in the gliding of the vertebrae, which squeezes the intervertebral discs to one side to produce a herniation or bulge. This bulging or herniated disc may irritate or compress a major nerve emerging out of the vertebral column, resulting in excruciating backache or neurological symptoms (referred pain, numbness, tingling, loss of power in the limbs etc) – that darned 'slipped disc' again!

Just to illustrate how absurd the diagnosis of 'slipped disc' can be, I was on a flight from Delhi to London after one of my Indian trips with a group of my patients. Midway through the flight they paged for a doctor. I volunteered. It was a British Airways security officer stretched out on a First-Class bed with excruciating back-ache. He had had food poisoning in Dhaka (Bangladesh) and been put on heavy antibiotics for persistent diarrhoea and sickness. I examined him, and found him severely dehydrated (he couldn't keep the water down and was therefore sick) with excruciating pain in the lumbar (kidney) region. I wanted to put him on a drip but the gentleman refused to have it. He found my diagnosis very strange (obviously he didn't trust me). His belief was that he had slipped a disc caused by violent sickness when he bent over the toilet unit. I couldn't help him so I requested the supervisor to arrange for an ambulance at Heathrow and to tell the paramedic there to put him on the drip anyway. I was quite confident (conviction comes from experience) that rehy-dration therapy would have helped a lot. A continuous pain like that in the lower mid-back area in all postural positions could not be disc-related. Moreover, the food-poisoning and the intake of heavy antibiotics (which can sometimes cause pain in the kidneys) completes the story and my logical deduction.

Chapter 6

Physiological Analysis of Posture

Keeping the Spine Erect

There are up to six layers of muscles around the spine, which can be roughly divided into (i) superficial and (ii) deep layers. The superficial or outer layer nearest the surface consists of extensors, which means these muscles pull the upper body backwards to keep it erect. Because they are credited with keeping it erect, they are called, in conventional medical terminology, 'erector spinae'. However, as we discovered in Chapter 4, the muscles that pull the body backwards, do not play a major role in keeping the spine erect. The true 'erector spinae' muscles are different from those science describes in medical textbooks. Inside these powerful superficial 'erector spinae' muscles are different muscle fibres that act as the true erector of the spine. The muscles that science has described as 'erector spinae' should be called 'dorsal extensor muscles' as these muscle fibres pull the body back into an erect position and then the true 'erector spinae' take over.

The bulk of the body's weight, as mentioned earlier, is in front of the spine. This weight is derived from such organs as the heart, lungs, liver, kidneys, intestines, uterus, bladder etc. Behind the spine there is only muscle and the skin. Thus, in order to prevent the body from stooping over to the front, the back muscles pull the spine back into an erect position, where another group of muscles take over to keep the body erect. When you carry a heavy weight in your hands you can feel the tendency in the lumbar and other muscles at the back to pull you back to prevent you bending forward too much. As mentioned earlier, even the lumbar curvature changes to adjust the body's posture to cope with the situation created by a heavy weight in front of the spine.

A similar situation can arise from excess weight gain. The fat deposit in the abdomen and the 'belly' can create a constant strain on the back muscles, which ultimately leads to chronic backache.

Bending

The extensors of the back (I will avoid calling them 'erector spinae' for the reasons I have given above) are of different lengths. Some originate at the base of the skull and end at the level of the upper thoracic vertebrae. These muscles, known as 'semi-spinalis capitis', can pull the head back as they shrink. Other muscles originate at the level of the upper back and end on the sacrum at the base of the spine. These muscles, known as 'sacrospinalis', can bend the thoracic spine back. If the 'semi-spinalis capitis' and 'sacrospinalis' act together, as in the case of a gymnast trying to arch the body back in order to touch the floor with her hands, the entire spine will extend or bend backward.

Thus Nature has given us muscles of different lengths to cater for the varying degrees of shrinkage required to carry out a function. If slight bending is required the short back muscles will shrink and if the entire spine is expected to bend backwards, the entire muscles running the length of the spine will shrink. The varying lengths of muscles allow both fine and gross movements of the spine.

If one side of the extensor muscles on the spine shrinks the spine will bend towards that side laterally. If both sides shrink then the spine will bend backward. Similarly, there are anterior (frontal) groups of spinal muscles, located in front of the spine. These are called 'flexor muscles' (opposite of 'extensors'). There are very few flexor muscles in front of the spine except in the neck and lumbar regions. This is so because many of the large trunk muscles, like the abdominal muscles in front of the body, when shrinking bend the spine forward by themselves. The neck has many short and long flexors (known as 'longus coli' and 'longus capitis') which enable the head and neck to bend forward. The lumbar region has a powerful group of flexors known as 'quadratus lumborum' which facilitate such movements as sit-ups and bending the spine forward so that the forehead can touch the front of the thighs or kneecap. There are no anterior flexor muscles in the thoracic area as the chest houses vital organs (the heart and lungs) and bending forward could damage blood vessels and these organs.

The neck has many different types of muscle varying in size and direction. This is because the head and neck have to move in all different directions. Thus rotation of the head to one side is carried out by sternocleidomastoid, longus capitis etc on the same side. Tilting the head sideways is enabled by the anterior scalene, longus coli etc on the desired side. All these muscles coordinate with each other to produce synchronic movement of the head. A perfect example of such fine movements can be seen in 'Bharatnatyan', an Indian classical dance form where the exponent carries out perfectly coordinated movements of the head and neck, resulting in the head moving sideways without tilting.

Deep Layer of Spinal Muscle

The deep muscles of the spine, often known as intrinsic or para-vertebral muscles, interconnect and stabilise the vertebrae. They are relatively short muscles (up to 60 of them) that are either attached to adjacent vertebrae or cross one vertebra and are attached to the one following it (see Figure on page 72). In various combinations, their shrinkage produces slight extension or rotation of the spinal column. Their main function is to stabilise adjacent vertebrae and to make delicate adjustments to the position of individual vertebrae. Thus if the spinal column has rotated and then returned to its normal position, the chances are that some vertebrae may not have returned to their perfect aligned position. Since the vertebrae have to be in perfect alignment in order to maintain the body's erect posture, the smaller but deep muscles of the spine play an important role in returning them to their final destination.

These muscles are thus vital in fine-tuning the spinal alignment. Injury to these delicate muscles, through injury or bad posture, can hinder natural alignment of the

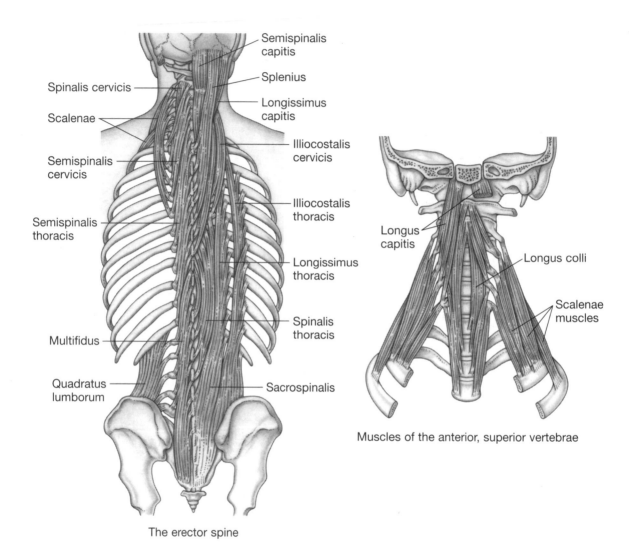

Semispinalis
capitis

Spinalis cervicis

Splenius

Scalenae

Longissimus
capitis

Semispinalis
cervicis

Illiocostalis
cervicis

Illiocostalis
thoracis

Semispinalis
thoracis

Longus
capitis

Longus colli

Longissimus
thoracis

Scalenae
muscles

Multifidus

Spinalis
thoracis

Quadratus
lumborum

Sacrospinalis

Muscles of the anterior, superior vertebrae

The erector spine

vertebrae. As we will see later, this disalignment of vertebra(e) can cause abnormal pressure on the disc(s) and cause it/them to bulge or even herniate. This can cause compression of nerves, producing pain and other neurological symptoms like tingling, numbness etc. Moreover, from my experience, it is these delicate muscles that, when injured, produce more complications of the spine than the injury of strong superficial muscles. Posture adjustment is a fine matter and tough muscles can play only a small role. The delicate deep muscles of the spine play a more important role in the genesis of backache and its cure. Their weakness may cause backache and their strengthening may improve or prevent the condition.

Functions of Spinal Muscles

There are many functions of the spinal muscles but they fall into two main groups:

 1

Voluntarily controlled functions. These are:

a   movements like bending, rotating, and many other complicated actions

b   lifting, carrying (on the back), pushing etc (here muscles tighten up to increase power before moving).

 2

Involuntarily (subconscious) controlled functions. These include:

a   maintaining tone of muscles

b   maintaining erect posture

c   controlling balance.

The functions that are voluntarily controlled are relatively easy to understand. Muscles shrink, producing movements. As they do that they tighten up and therefore can bear weight.

Involuntarily controlled functions of spinal muscles need some logical understanding. Some facts are known about the subconscious control of the body but there is a lot that is still unknown. I will do my best to explain in simple terms how muscles control posture and tone driven by the subconscious brain and the spinal cord.

Reflexes

First I must explain what reflexes are. A reflex is a reaction of the body to certain changes that take place within the body. Let us see how in the following examples:

1

You touch something hot and automatically the hand is snatched away to prevent the fingers from getting burned. The nerve endings on the fingertips that feel heat send impulses via sensory nerves to the spine where a 'process centre' or 'analysing centre' in the brain promptly sends commands to the muscles via motor nerves to withdraw the hand immediately. This path from fingertips to the spine to the muscles of the arm is a reflex. It is almost like the rays of the sun being reflected by a mirror on to the wall.

2

You feel cold and the body responds to it in a certain way: you shiver to generate more body heat; you get goose pimples to trap a layer of air between 'raised hair' on the skin to prevent heat loss from its surface; your body mobilises reserve glucose and fat to release more fuel to generate heat. All these different responses (involuntary) come about because of the stimulation of cold 'receptors' or nerve endings on the skin. These receptors send messages to the subconscious brain which processes the information before sending commands to the autonomous (involuntary) nerve centres to shiver, create 'goose bumps' and release glucose. This is a complex reflex with a series of reactions to a single stimulus (cold).

3

A doctor uses a patellar hammer to strike the tendon below the kneecap and almost instantly the knee jerks. This is a common reflex tested by doctors on a routine examination. They strike on the thick tendon below the kneecap, stretching it suddenly. This in turn leads to sudden stretching of the muscle fibres of the quadriceps, the powerful thigh muscles. The special receptors in the muscle fibres send a message to the spinal cord where it is processed or analysed instantly before relaying it to the motor (movement) centres in the spine, which command the muscle fibres of the quadriceps to shrink immediately, producing the 'jerk'. This reflex is known as a stretch reflex.

Stretch reflex is the main modus operandi of posture control. Let us examine this closely to understand this phenomenon. Embedded in the muscle fibres are special structures called 'spindles'. These spindles have fibres that are activated by proprio-receptors or nerve endings that perceive or sense pressure. As soon as the stretching takes place, these spindles flatten out stimulating the special receptors or muscle endings. This results in an instant transfer of messages to the spinal cord, where they are reflected back to the muscle fibres around the spindles. As soon as that happens the fibres contract and the entire muscle shortens, thus completing the reflex.

When a person leans forward, the spindles in the muscles of the calves, hamstrings and the glutens (seat muscles) and spine are stretched. This results in their shrinking and the body is pulled back into an erect position. Similarly when a person leans back, the spindles of the muscles of the skin, quadriceps, abdomen and other anterior muscles get stretched. This produces a stretch reflex resulting in these muscles shrinking to pull the body forward, thus reinstating the balanced erect position. Stretch reflexes, therefore, pull the body backwards and forward as and when it is necessary to adjust the body's posture to maintain an erect position. All these happen without the participation of the conscious brain. Since they are reflexes, these reactions are spontaneous and automatic (involuntary).

In the body, however, more complex reflexes take place to maintain the balanced erect position. For example, it is not only the forward and backward movements that maintain the erect position, there are lateral (sideways) movements too that need to be coordinated. The stretch reflex explains the basic mechanism by which posture is maintained, although the complexity of reactions or movements is very intricate.

When a person trips on the street, a series of quick reflex movements are automatically put into action to prevent the body from falling and injuring itself. Most of these movements are involuntarily and only a few quick response voluntary movements are made to react to this emergency situation. A marvellous part of this reflex action is that in an open space the reflex is entirely one of regaining balance, while if there is a wall or a post handy the arms will involuntarily shoot out for support. Similarly during walking, jogging, working in an erect position and in sports activities, a whole series of reflexes (involuntarily movements) and voluntary movements maintain the posture of the body. In the above situations, the posture changes all the time and therefore it is up to the spinal muscles to shrink, relax and extend to keep the spine erect in these altered positions of the body.

Role of Reflexes in Posture

As mentioned earlier, the muscle fibres responsible for keeping the spine and the body erect extend upwards creating an anti-gravitational force. This force is powerful enough to support the weight of the body as well as to stretch the spine upwards. In a horizontal position such stretching is also possible and we took this into account when our yoga exercises were derived for treatment of back problems. In the horizontal or resting position the muscle extension is less powerful as it does not have the additional task of supporting the weight of the body. It seems obvious, logically speaking, that the 'weight-bearing' muscle fibres switch into action only when they face the gravitational force (known as 'body weight'). This force acting downwards towards the centre of the earth puts stress on the weight-bearing muscle fibres and triggers off a reflex action that makes them extend upwards counteracting the body weight by anti-gravitational force, in particular taking pressure off the discs.

The capacity to stretch upwards, given to the spinal and other muscles responsible for keeping the body erect (such as the legs, thigh, calves, shin), is phenomenal. Thus, one can lift a heavy weight, as weightlifters do, and these muscles will co-operate up to a point depending on their training and endurance. There is a limit to how much weight these muscles can support before damaging the body (tendons, joints, discs etc). Extra weight on the body requires extra power in the muscles as the anti-gravitational force created must support this weight to prevent damage to the body. That is why sudden weight gain without exercises or training of posture muscles can cause problems in the lower back, hip and knee joints. The muscles that create the anti-gravitational force are compelled to create additional power and maintain it all the time as weight gain is a constant factor.

Jumping

Imagine somebody jumping down to the ground from a certain height. The shock of the fall is immediately absorbed by the muscles of the spine and legs. The spring-like action created by bent ankles, knees and hip joints also participates in the shock absorption. The main role, however, is performed by muscles that switch into action through reflexes and involuntary movements. Depending on the height of the fall, the impact can be substantial and yet the muscles and bones absorb it without any consequence whatsoever. The quick reflexes and synchronised coordination of muscle fibres at the subconscious level achieves this.

When a person jumps down, the muscles of the spine, those that are involved in keeping the spine erect, begin to react synchronically as soon as the feet hit the ground. They stretch upward to create a rapid response and absorb the shock. This sudden genesis of anti-gravitational force reduces the effect of impact on the ground. This force is a gift of Nature as an impact with body weight on the ground can crush joints, bones and certainly vertebral discs. This force prevents injuries to the delicate tissues of the body. If however the fall is from a great height or the body is very heavy or the muscles are not strong enough to create the anti-gravitational thrust at the moment of impact, then injuries to the various structures mentioned above are inevitable. Imagine, though, if the reflex were achieved, as science would have us believe, by the superficial muscles contracting like guy ropes to keep the body erect, how much extra pressure there would be on the discs. Parachutists would never survive. Thank goodness Nature designed us better than that!

Stress

We must consider another factor that creates the upward thrust or anti-gravitational force responsible for keeping the spine erect. When muscles 'contract', they shrink. In other words the muscle fibres slide into each other producing the shortening of the muscle length, which is misleadingly termed 'contraction'. When the muscles are relaxed the muscle fibres return to their normal positions, sliding away from each other. Thus when muscles are tensed they are shorter in length than when they are relaxed. Stress causes increase in tone of muscles as the fibres increase in tension. In a state of relaxation the muscles lengthen as the fibres return to the normal position. Thus in stressful situations, the spinal muscles are tensed and the chances of disc compression increase. In a relaxed state of mind, the muscles return to their normal length, thus facilitating decompression of discs. This can explain why tensed people get backache. Actors, however, are taught to relax totally when they fall on stage to avoid injury.

Summary

To sum up what has been said, it is clear that the erect posture of man is maintained by the muscle fibres of the spinal and leg muscles and these are different from those that control movement or carry weight. These muscle fibres extend upwards creating an anti-gravitational force or upward thrust that keeps the body erect. Moreover, these muscle fibres are involuntarily controlled but can be adjusted by the conscious brain to a certain degree. Finally, the more powerful the upward thrust, the less the compression of discs and other joint surfaces that participate in weight-bearing.

The body, in its effort to stay erect, has empowered the muscles of the spine to counteract the weight of the vital organs in front of it (lungs, liver, heart, intestines etc) by continuously pulling back and preventing the body from stooping over. This is happening involuntarily all the time when one sits or stands erect.

Chapter 7

Care of the Spine
to Prevent Disorders

It is crucial to take care of the spine for general health. I gave detailed advice on keeping healthy in my earlier book *The Integrated Health Bible*. In brief, I recommended adopting a Lifestyle Programme based on moderation and variety supported by diet, massage and exercise. In particular I recommended massage and exercises for the spine, the latter including specific yoga exercises, swimming and walking. The significance of the yoga exercises is expanded in this book, since I hope I have made it clear that it is so much more important for the back to develop and tone up the posture-maintaining muscles than to work away at the lifting and carrying muscles so emphasised in manuals and gymnasia. The posture-maintaining muscles are deep and hard to access. Even normal massage does not have ready access to them. The Thai type of massage, which develops and tones through stretching, can work on them and this is also taken into account in yoga.

I also gave a list of the benefits of walking and would like to emphasise one of them here – it improves posture. Study of reflexes shows that repetitive exercises will contribute little to this vital function. Common sense, however, tells us that to walk over uneven ground will bring the reflexes into play constantly. Even stepping over a sleeping dog, will do more good to your posture than several minutes of repetitive aerobic exercises because it makes the reflexes do what they are supposed to do – meet the unexpected. In this chapter, therefore, I will concentrate on general care of the spine, from birth, or before, to old age, with particular emphasis on the posture-maintaining muscles.

Care During Pregnancy

Though it is important to treat the spine as a whole, for the sake of clarity I will consider different parts of it separately. Prevention of injuries and other complications of the cervical spine is a complex matter and is vital because of its impact on the nutrition of the subconscious brain. The process should start at a child's conception. A good healthy diet, plus vitamins and folic acid which are essential for the prevention of spina bifida, for the mother with regular gentle exercises like therapeutic yoga ensures healthy pregnancy with good development of the foetus.

The diet should exclude alcohol, coffee, excess refined sugar, yeast products, canned or preserved products, cheese, very spicy food, excess salt, mushrooms, excess garlic and ginger etc. These substances either 'excite' the central nervous system (coffee, alcohol, excess garlic or ginger) or are toxic for the pregnancy (mushrooms, preservatives). Excess yeast and sugar may produce flatulence, which can cause discomfort and pain in the abdomen.

Food should be well cooked to make it easily digestible. It should be fresh and palatable. The diet of a pregnant woman should contain sufficient amounts of protein, fruits, fresh vegetables, pomegranate, spinach, salad, sprouts, soaked (overnight) almonds, carrot juice etc. The protein ensures healthy development of the foetus and spinach, pomegranates and soaked almonds help blood synthesis by supplementing iron and protein. Dinner should be light, as heavy foods may cause discomfort at night in bed. Lunch should be the main meal.

A pregnant woman should drink plenty of water and take an afternoon nap. She should avoid late nights and undue exertion. Lifting of heavy weights, vigorous exercises, 'energetic' dances, horse riding, motorbike rides and standing for long hours are not advisable. If possible she should take the last trimester off on maternity leave (three months before the expected time of delivery). Frequent air travel, long journeys resulting in jet-lag syndrome and sea journeys (motion sickness) are also not advised.

Posture in pregnancy

Try and walk without exaggerating the lower back arch and don't turn the feet out. Keep them straight when walking. This helps to keep the weight off the front bones (femur) of the legs thereby reducing strain on the spine. Keep kneed slightly bent and lengthen the spine upwards. Release the lower part of your spine (sacrum) by lengthening it, let it 'drop' down; your pelvis will automatically lift up and position itself below the abdomen. You will also be carrying your baby closer to yourself, closer to the spine.

Regular therapeutic yoga is extremely beneficial for relaxation, circulation and proper development of labour muscles. The breathing exercises help to de-stress the mother and the foetus. Over the page are some examples of the exercises and yogic postures advisable for pregnant women.

Yoga Exercises

Child pose or pawan mukt

sometimes called half-embryo or wind-releasing pose.

● Breathe in, bring your right knee to your chest, keep the left leg straight.

● Breathe out slowly, bringing your forehead to touch your knee.

● Lower your head to the floor slowly, keeping your chin towards your neck and breathing in.

● Breath out, relax arms and straighten leg.

● Repeat this with your other leg.

● Do this five times with each leg.

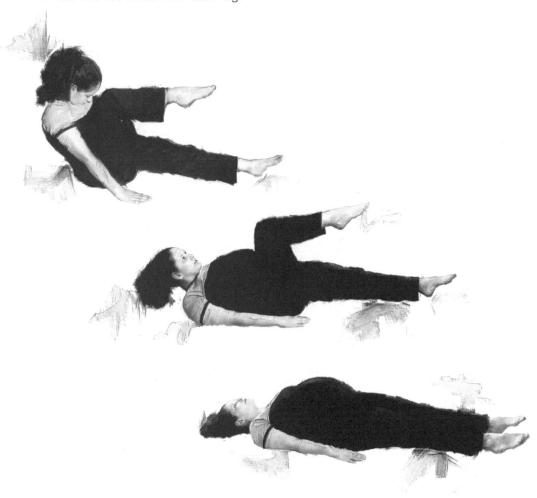

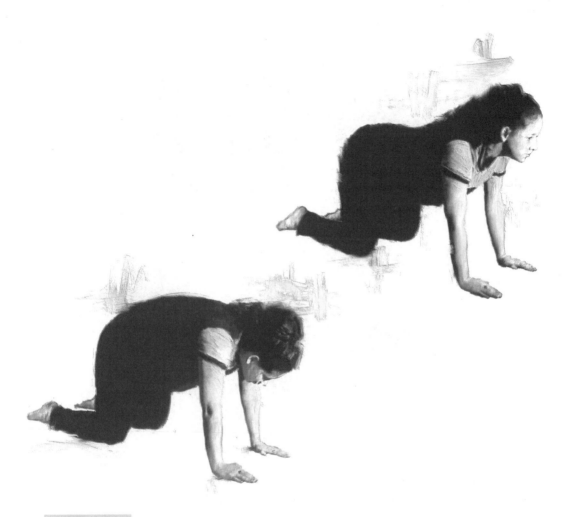

Bilikasana·

- Go forward onto all fours – hands are placed below the shoulders and knees below hips.
- Breathe out and arch up the spine by pulling up from the arms and shoulders and contracting the stomach muscles look down.
- Slowly arch down the spine on breathing in, pulling away shoulders from the neck and stretching neck forwards and not up.
- Repeat five times.

This posture, as well as safely loosening up the spine, is extremely beneficial for returning the uterus to the correct position after childbirth. It can be does as an ante-natal or post-natal exercise.

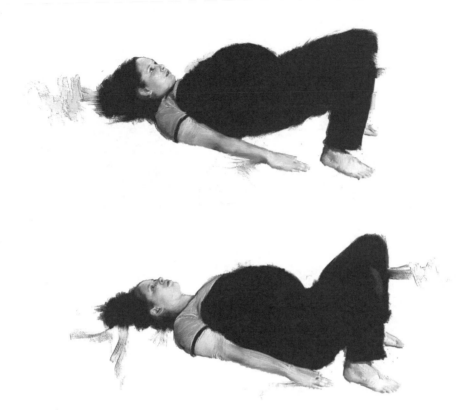

Setubandhasana (bridge)

- Lie down on your back and relax the whole spine
- Keep your arms by your sides, ankles below your knees, hip-distance apart.
- Feel the waist against the floor on breathing out and lift up your back without jolting.
- Keep your legs steady by keeping the knees above the ankles and pushing heels down to the ground.
- Push down on the hands to steady the posture.
- Stretch the neck away from the shoulders by lowering the chin towards the chest – take a deep breath as you do this.
- Lower the back slowly, feeling each vertebra of the spine on the floor and relax the feet, arms and spine.
- Repeat two times. Straighten your legs.

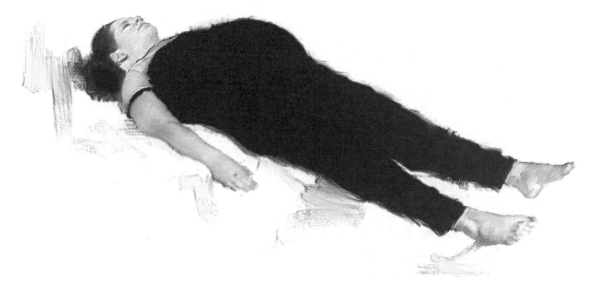

Shavasana

(see page 114)

Care of the Newborn

It is hoped that the above measures would help normal delivery of the baby. The care for the newborn becomes very important for the future development of the body. The baby comes out through the tensed birth canal which, even in its dilated state, is smaller in size than the baby's head and the rest of the body. A very rapid birth can cause as much damage as an extremely laborious and slow one. If the contractions are right, with the right duration and power, the baby will inch its way through the canal safely and less traumatically. Personal care of oneself during pregnancy increases the chances of synchronisation of all the events of delivery.

Massage of the newborn is an art. For thousands of years the midwives of India (known as 'Dais') have been doing it in their own special way. There used to be a dedicated school, in the ancient city of Benares, that trained such Dais.

A Dai takes care of the mother and child for forty days after the delivery. The mother is massaged for her comfort and therapy. The various techniques used help her to get rid of fatigue, swellings in the body, excess cellulite on the body (women would think all cellulite was 'excess'), stretch marks on the abdomen, and she is helped to maintain a steady flow of milk for the baby.

Traditionally, the baby gets its first massage when it is five days old. That is when it is first bathed in water with a little salt and aqueous solution of the Neem leaves (for their antiseptic properties). Mustard oil or ghee (clarified butter) is used for massage. Even though mustard has a pungent smell it has many therapeutic properties and amongst them is its ability to warm up the muscles by drawing in more blood.

The baby is gently massaged all over with emphasis on the neck and shoulder area. It is placed on a mat, but surrounded by the legs of the Dai, with the head closer to her ankles, and massaged. These gentle but healing strokes soothe the most irritable of all babies and, even though they may struggle in the beginning, they later become very calm, often falling asleep. After the massage, the baby is put out to lie and soak in the morning sun, first on the back and then on the stomach for a few minutes. After this it is bathed and wrapped up warm. The wrapping of the baby in a clean cotton cloth is in itself an art. The spine, right up to the neck, is maintained in a straight alignment with the help of the cloth. This ritualistic therapy of the mother and child goes on for 40 days and it gives the baby's musculo-skeletal system the best chance to rectify the trauma of birth and help it to develop.

Unfortunately, this tradition is fast dying in India, like so many other useful and sensible things. The urge to be modern is so strong that one by one that country is shedding all its traditional values and practices.

Massage of the baby can be done quite safely by the mother, or her helper, if she has one. At the Integrated Medical Centre we have developed an oil, which we simply call 'Baby/Junior Massage Oil', containing a base oil with mustard, avocado and sesame. A few drops of Eucalyptus, lavender and camomile oils can also be added before massage. The baby can be gently massaged all over the body. It should be massaged with the thumb and the index finger on either side.

This massage should be done daily for a month and then a couple of times a week for two more months. This will ensure proper development of the baby, strengthening the muscles and the bones. In an overwhelming majority of cases, the baby remains calm and relaxed, without any signs of colds or infections. Such babies raise their heads, sit, crawl, and walk at the right time, indicating a healthy development.

When breastfeeding the baby, it should be comfortably positioned in cradled arms. If it is breast-fed in bed, the mother should change breasts and the side on which she lies. Thus, when feeding with the left breast the mother should be to the right side of the baby and vice versa. This will prevent the baby from lying on one side all the time. However inconvenient this may be, it is important to ensure that the baby lies on both sides an equal number of times when breastfeeding or when sleeping in its cot.

Bedtime massage is a good practice for the developing child. Ideally, this should be carried out till three years of age about twice a week. This will ensure sound sleep and a well-balanced physical body. The neck and the spine will then grow perfectly normally. Massage has a hands-on healing effect, especially if the parents do it. They naturally have a strong bond with the baby and parents need to pass on this energy and warmth to their offspring. Dogs or animals in the wild would lick and nuzzle their cubs for precisely the same reason. Finally, massage done by parents develops a very healthy relationship between the parents and their child. This touching and caring can achieve far more than just the occasional hug or kiss.

Growing Up

As the child grows up, it falls often and hurts itself. In such times it is essential to massage the spine and neck for a few days even though the spine does not obviously seem to be affected. The fragile spine can take the shock of any fall or jerk and register it, leaving varying magnitudes of imbalances in it.

The pillow used in bed is a very important factor in the care of the neck and prevention of complications in the future. Children usually sleep on their sides cuddled up, so a medium-size pillow is more suitable, as the distance between the shoulder and the neck should be taken into account. If it sleeps on its back then a thinner pillow is required. As the child grows, attention should be paid to this and pillow sizes should be adjusted to the growth of the child. The rule is 'the thinner the pillow, the better'.

The child should be discouraged from sleeping or reading or watching TV on its stomach for long periods of time. In bed, the child should sit up to read and not get into the habit of lying down to read. All these put strain on the neck. Posture when sitting is important. Even as a child one should always sit with the thighs horizontal. If you buy him a table and chair when a toddler, and he is still using this at the age of 12 he will be sure to develop bad postural habits. Children's furniture should be adjustable. The same thing applies to shoes. Children grow out of their shoes then continue to wear them, which distorts their feet and hence their posture.

Parents should ask children about any falls or injuries at school. If they have had any, a simple examination of the neck should be carried out. The neck, being fragile, takes 'shock waves' of a fall more readily and can become disaligned. A simple manual examination will reveal any defect, as it would always hurt when the trauma is 'registered'. Massage of that area will resolve the problem in most cases.

If the child plays vigorous games such as rugby, where the chances of injury to the neck greatly increase, professional help from a person who knows the Ali Technique or a chiropractor or osteopath who deals with children, should be sought. It is best to have a quarterly checkup in any case, if the child plays vigorous games or is accident-prone at other times.

Computers and video games seem to be causing neck injuries (many undetected) in epidemic proportions. It is such an addictive pastime that children find it difficult to get away from it. Although it is ideal for parents, as they get spared from being bothered all the time with questions and demands, one should take adequate precautions that the child rests from it periodically. The excitement, the posture and the immobility caused by these gadgets result in many physical and psychological problems. Seizures from these games have been recognised by some manufacturers and they warn parents, in small print, about these dangers.

It is so difficult to monitor all the developmental problems a child goes through, that it becomes almost impossible to correct them. Therefore it is advisable to give periodic correctional therapy and encourage them to do the various yogic exercises recommended in this book. These are best done in schools and can be incorporated into the physical training classes, which are part of the school curriculum anyway. Schools should take part in the physical development of the children. For example, children nowadays are growing very tall and quickly, so the classroom furniture should be adjusted to this growing demand. Desks and chairs should not all be of standard size but should be designed to take into account the varying heights of pupils. Boarding schools in particular should pay more attention to these matters, just as should parents of children who stay at home. Bad posture, coupled with poorly designed furniture, can definitely affect the spines of growing children.

Nutritional matters should also be taken into account for the development of the spine. Firstly, foods that are canned, preserved and pre-cooked do have reduced nutritional value. Secondly, fast foods should be avoided as far as possible. The application of common and human sense in food matters is of utmost importance. The breaking up of family values and the traditional parent/child relationships has led to the near extinction of the culture of cooking family meals, and of eating habits that used to exist in the good old days. Lack of time and financial demands have led to the culture of convenience cooking. There is no reason why breakfast and dinner cannot be healthy and delicious. Special attention must be given to fast-growing children's demand for calcium. Their 'growing pains' should be signals for a change in their eating habits. In the teenage period, bad nutrition and posture are the two most common factors that cause poor development of the spine. Accidents and traumas are simply secondary causes, as a strong spine can take the shock of a trauma more easily.

General Care of the Adult Spine

In today's world, life has become very compacted. The dilemmas, the deadlines and the human interaction have led to high levels of stress. Most people exist rather than live. Poor nutrition, heavy workload, lack of exercise, lack of sound sleep, bad posture and stress are the constant physical and mental traumas the body faces on a regular basis. It is therefore essential to look into these factors to prevent illness and maintain well-being.

Here are some factors that need to be looked into, for the maintenance of the neck and the rest of the spine:

Sleep

It is very important to have good quality sleep at night. It is during sleep that the body gets an opportunity to build, repair and regenerate energy. Firstly, one should allow plenty of time for sleep to take place. Late nights and long working hours obviously cut into the recommended sleeping time, which is approximately seven hours for an adult. Secondly, one should allow enough time to unwind before falling asleep. A short walk helps enormously. Using fatigue as an excuse to go to bed immediately will result in waking up very early (around 3–4am) when the fatigue wears off and the day hormones begin to accumulate in the blood. A bit of reading, talking with the family to exchange each other's daily experiences, watching a pleasant (not disturbing) programme or film on TV or listening to music are a few common tips to help the body and mind relax. Brief breathing exercises and stretching at bedtime help this tremendously.

I strongly advise everyone to use the lunch break to take a brief nap if it is at all possible. The neck and the spine demand rest from time to time. Animals do it and, in my opinion, humans should follow this natural example. In some countries, the practice of an afternoon break (siesta) is traditional and highly beneficial. A break in the afternoon, shortly after lunch, is the best prevention of neck and spinal complications.

Mechanical strain on the neck (Repetitive Strain Injury)

Computers have become the single most hazardous working tool humans have, especially when used excessively. As one of my old teachers once said: 'Computers will ruin human beings one day.' To that I add, 'Computers will become a noose around the neck of human kind – literally.' The damage it causes to the neck and the complications that arise out of that are unbelievable. It used to be the screen that was blamed for the fatigue, blurred vision, irritability, insomnia, headaches, dizziness etc so there was an industry built up for screen filters which in general had little or no effect. Staring at a screen in a fixed position, however, contradicts the very principle of the existence of the neck. Nature has given the neck the extraordinary function to move in all directions and that is why it is structured differently from the rest of the body. The neck is meant to move and not be fixed. On top of that the neck muscles are tightened by stress, the stress of reading from the screen, writing, analysing, thinking and making decisions all at the same time.

When computers were first introduced into offices, the general impression that was created was that they would make the employees' work easier and more convenient so that they would do their work more efficiently and have plenty of free time to themselves. Unfortunately, the opposite has happened and people have ended up doing more work and straining their neck and arms. To counteract this, the computer industry came up with a model that would automatically switch off every two hours so that the user could take a break. Unfortunately, this model did not become popular.

When using computers to excess you soon get degeneration of the discs – degeneration of the joints takes place much later. And it can be prevented. If you use a computer for more than six hours at a time you should try regularly, at least every other day, to massage the neck area and I would suggest that you yourself massage the jaws, the temples and the neck muscles. You have to do it on a regular basis. There is no way of avoiding this. Otherwise the problem just accumulates. People get panic attacks, terrific neck tension, they get tremendously stressed, all because of the tightening of the neck. Even the vertebral arteries, which feed the subconscious brain, can become restricted, causing what has come to be known in my clinic as the Ali Syndrome (see also page 173). This is a recognisable set of symptoms including fatigue, blurred vision, dizziness, nausea, short-term memory loss, confusion and lack of verbal expression, tinnitus, autoimmune disorders, loss of libido, menstrual dysfunctions in women, depression, disturbed sleep, craving for sugar, hyperventilation and palpitations, burning mouth syndrome, mood swings, allergies, poor immune system with frequent coughs and colds, impotence ... Need I go on? You don't want it, do you?

If you work at a computer you should take preventive action all the time. Computer neck ache is not usually the nerve impingement type or the more usual spondilitis type of ache. It is more muscular. When your neck is moving the flow of blood is good, but in a static, spasmodic or tensed state the circulation is poor. You then get neck tension, which is basically of the lactic acid type. Very often if you swim or do a little exercise it gets dispersed and the pain goes away. But you have to treat it or prevent it, working on focal areas, because sometimes it cannot release the tension on its own and can result in insomnia-related neck ache. This is a similar type of thing. You toss around and each time you think of anything stressful the neck muscles go into a continuous repetitive tightness.

In this connection I ought to mention Repetitive Strain Injury or overuse syndrome. Using the same muscles to work continuously on the keyboard combined with the strain on the neck and arm muscles has created a new disease, RSI. Industrial tribunals are dealing with thousands of claimants whose lives have been ruined by overuse of computers. Drivers and people doing desk jobs for long hours face similar problems. Their head is fixed in one position for a long time while the arm muscles are taut as they carry out the job.

Unless care is taken to metabolise the lactic acid (a by-product formed in the muscles from strenuous and prolonged contractions) and to reduce the strain on the ligaments, inflammation or injury is bound to take place. A sum total of these minor injuries leads to loss of function of the part of the body involved.

Frequent Flying

Flying is one of the greatest hazards of the international business community. Long-hand air travel across several time zones puts tremendous strain on the body and mind. Each hour of flight is like a day's laborious work so if one does a seven-hour flight one has done enough work for a week, especially if it is across the meridians and time zones.

The most common symptoms of the post-flight period, such as headaches, dizziness, nausea, fatigue, palpitations, lack of concentration etc, are connected, as I have said, with neck problems. That is why the strain in the neck and back is so obvious after each long flight. Drinking water, sleeping, walking up and down the aisle and doing the exercises recommended in the airline magazine or entertainment programme rarely make much difference on long-haul flights.

Travel sickness, a kind of anxiety that builds up before air travel, is part of the same problem. The strain of travel begins well before the flying takes place. Some airlines provide limousine services, easy check-in and pre-flight comfort (massages, pedicure etc) for their business and First Class passengers to cater to these needs. Post-flight lounges of some airlines also look into the comfort and pampering of high-fare-paying passengers. Economy travellers bear the full brunt of the hazards of flying, from uncomfortable seats to cramped cabins. The strain of air travel is well accepted and known in extreme cases to be lethal, as can be seen from the publicity on DVT (Deep Vein Thrombosis), but it is considered to be a price people have to pay for travelling. Reduced oxygen level in the cabin (deliberately imposed to reduce costs) can cause muscle ache and the accumulation of lactic acid in the body. Crew members have to take a couple of days off just to get over the strain. They would be sick and too tired to function otherwise. In addition, the cabin crew work during flights – lifting, carrying, pushing trolleys etc. They get terrible back-aches. Take-offs and landings and their potential risks act on the subconscious mind and produce their own range of shocks to the system. Also, no journey starts and finishes on the aircraft, there are often hours of hassle at each end to add on to the strain of air travel. Furthermore, the extra security measures adopted since 11 September 2001 add to this stress for everyone.

Business travellers face additional problems after the flights. Different hotel beds with varying sizes of pillows and firmness of beds cause obvious damage to the neck and spine. Pillows and beds are personal comforts or props that people get used to, and so, when they change them often, there is likely to be damage to the neck and back. Most air travellers suffer from neck and back problems. They get stressed out after doing it for a while. The effects of this stress are reflected on their faces. They look tired and age very quickly. In the days before the crew members' union, stewards and stewardesses were renewed frequently to keep fresh-looking staff on board. It is not surprising why one sees so many tired-looking faces on flights. In my opinion cabin crew members should retire at 40 and take up ground jobs.

Jet lag is another major complication of long-haul flights. This takes a lot out of a person. Adjusting to time zones all the time is a great strain on the system as a whole. Transit can be an extra strain, but in some airports, such as Bangkok, a transit break can be turned to advantage by taking a massage while waiting. This can undo hours of damage on the flight.

Importance of Posture

Posture is determined by (a) the state of the spine and (b) the strain and stress that the person faces. Apart from diseases of the spine (scoliosis, osteoarthritis, disc problems), bad posture can lead to a lot of spinal problems, not the least of which I mentioned earlier, namely that it can engage the superficial spinal muscles permanently in maintaining the bad posture, letting the deep muscles wither and placing continuous excess pressure on the discs through the guy rope effect. Education or maintenance through the Alexander Technique, Pilates and yoga is very important. Only a conscientious effort to maintain the posture at work and rest can eliminate all the problems related to posture.

Sometimes posture is determined by one's personality reflected through the subconscious. Opposite are some examples:

Forward-thinking
Always ahead of everybody

Proud
Confident

Insecure
Lack of confidence, scared

Sometimes, the posture changes in the growing phase. It is something one acquires. For example, teenage girls who are embarrassed about their large breasts bring the shoulders forward in an attempt to make them less conspicuous. This changes the shape of the neck and upper back.

Using too many pillows and sleeping on the stomach changes the shape of the neck and upper back, causing postural problems.

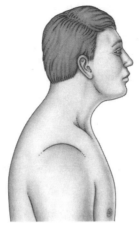

Forward-thinking
(fast-thinking, intense personality)

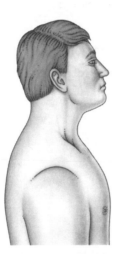

Proud
(proud, confident personality)

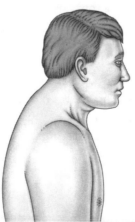

Insecure
(shy, timid, lack of confidence)

Postural defects alter the shape of the neck and the rest of the spine. These changes are reinforced by tight and fortified ligaments. The tendons at the end of muscles become taut and shortened with continuous spasms of muscles and postural abnormalities. The tightness of the ligaments (often heavily calcified) and shortening of the muscles, to alter posture permanently, makes it very difficult to treat diseases related to the neck.

Daniel, a 52-year-old, came to me with a deformed upper back and neck area due to previous postural problems. He suffered from chronic fatigue, tinnitus, dizziness and headaches. I found it extremely difficult to correct the faults in the cervical spine to produce a permanent relief to his symptoms because they had become so set.

After a session, he would feel all right for a week or so, and thereafter all the symptoms would return. Even though he follows the Regimen Therapy and does regular yoga exercises recommended to him, there has not been a permanent relief. Daniel is a case of someone who has let his condition deteriorate beyond redemption, while a degree of care in earlier life could have prevented it.

Trauma

Although it is not common to injure oneself in a routine way, every accident or fall leaves some signs of damage to the alignment of the spine and can be seen in the iris of the eye for years afterwards. The shock waves from a fall and the body's quick and almost involuntary response to control damage are mostly responsible for the changes in the alignment of the spine.

Sports like judo, karate, rugby, wrestling etc have obvious effects on the spine. In fact in ancient India, bone-setting (a form of massage-manipulative therapy) was part of the curriculum of a course in wrestling. So frequently did the wrestlers get injured that they had to be trained to help each other to rectify the dislocations, muscle and ligament injuries. The best bone-setters are the wrestlers themselves. Horse riding, jet-skiing, skiing, paragliding, gymnastics etc carry their own risk of injury. Sometimes it is not even the skill of the person that matters. Certain recreational activities like diving with an oxygen tank on the back can be very traumatic. The head has to be pushed back to its maximum to get a view ahead while swimming. After a period of time, this postural distortion can cause neck injury.

Some neck problems are iatrogenic (iatr – doctor, genic – caused by) – caused by the medical profession. Stress of dental treatment causing tension in the neck muscles followed by a period of unnatural positioning of the head and neck has been known to cause disalignment of the cervical vertebrae. During major surgeries, at the moment of intubation, when a thick breathing tube is inserted into the trachea through the mouth, the chances of misalignment of the cervical spine are high. Due to intravenous anaesthesia with muscle relaxants, which precedes this procedure, the muscles of the body and the neck are completely atonic and offer no resistance to any movement of the head and neck, even beyond its physiological range. Traction of the neck with heavy force has been known to cause injuries to the ligaments of the neck which later cause problems. Unqualified and manipulative therapists in training (physiotherapists, chiropractors, osteopaths) in their enthusiasm to experiment and do what they are not trained to do, often cause damage to the neck. I have treated several patients who have had iatrogenic injuries to the neck.

So how do we combat all these hazards faced by the spine? In the next chapter I will deal with the servicing and testing of the spine to keep it healthy.

Chapter **8**

Servicing the Spine

Neck tensions and spine-related problems are a regular feature in a person's life. Long working hours and stress cause sufficient damage to the spine, even in a routine way, to cause problems. Therefore, one has to service or look after it regularly. Dogs, cats and wild animals stretch and yawn every now and then to tone up their muscles. In fact some yoga poses mimic the movements of these animals. Most of the yoga asanas or poses have been taken from nature and objects surrounding human beings. Thus there are cat poses, lion poses, tree poses, plough poses, wheel poses etc.

The following recommendations have been derived from years of experience in dealing with problems of the neck.

Nutrition – Good Things

In the list of things that should be eaten, in that they will have a positively good effect on your back, pay attention to the following:

Muscles and bones need calcium

therefore it is advisable to eat a certain amount of protein, like eggs, fish, milk, yoghurt, etc. As mentioned earlier, it is the vitamin D present in animal fat which is more important than the actual consumption of calcium. We are always told to avoid animal fat, but to do so completely can be disastrous. The Integrated Health motto, moderation and variety, remains the key to good health. Vitamin D, so deficient in cold temperate climates with less sunshine, is essential to the absorption of calcium. It is synthesised by the skin when it is exposed to sunlight.

Muscles need potassium

for contraction and this has to be replenished after excessive strenuous work. Carrots and bananas are good for potassium.

Supplements like magnesium that relaxes muscles and B complex

counter stress and strain. They should be taken for two months at a time and given gaps of a month to prevent the body from getting used to them and reducing their therapeutic effect. The body has a remarkable capacity for adaptation and although we are well aware of this when adapting to hot or cold weather, the process is just as relevant to supplements, often rendering them useless if taken on a continuous basis.

Nutrition – Bad Things

The following foodstuffs are to be avoided in the diet:

Coffee

as it tenses up muscles and may cause insomnia.

Excess citric juices and acid-producing foodstuffs

like dry nuts (in excess), very spicy foods, deep-fried food, canned or preserved food (they contain citric acid as preservatives), white wine and champagne, excess alcohol and certain medicines (the aspirin group). These acid-forming foods change the alkalinity of blood and cause inflammation of ligaments and joint surfaces, and in particular the collagen fibres in these connective tissues are affected. In traditional medicine (Ayurveda, Unani) acid foods like lemon, vinegar, orange etc are banned from regular use, as a preventative measure. Of all the fruits of nature, the citric fruits cause maximum damage to the body while the orange growers promote the vitamin C content and its obvious benefits.

Vitamin C (ascorbic acid) is an excellent component of these fruits but citric acid, the main natural component present in these fruits, is not. It is the citric acid that causes all the harm to the body. Genetically modified oranges compete with each other by containing more citric acid, the sharp taste often being mistakenly associated with vitamin C. That is why some orange juices, even the freshly squeezed ones, are so acid that they are 'undrinkable'. Often they have to be gulped down with discomfort in the throat and teeth afterwards. The heartburn that may follow is often neglected because the orange-growing lobby says 'orange juice prevents disease'. Old varieties of oranges, as found in developing countries, are not so acid, because they were not modified or tampered with (to make them seedless or have more citric acid to taste more sharp). About twenty years ago, eating an orange was pleasurable, as the pulp was not so acidic, but nowadays it is often impossible to enjoy it, unless one loves acidic foods. By juicing oranges, one removes the fibrous part of the fruit. These fibres, or pith, are alkaline and Nature's own antidote to the very acid pulp (the principle being that bitter neutralises acid) and therefore, if one is very keen on oranges, one should only eat them and not juice them.

Satsumas, mandarins, and other sweeter varieties of the orange family, when eaten whole, do not produce the damage that orange juice does. Also, some pink varieties of grapefruit, which have that 'bitter after-taste', are well balanced and can be safely eaten. These are good fruits.

Excess red meat, and fatty foods

cause arthritic changes in the joints.

Refined sugar, chocolate and sweets

cause arthritic changes and should not be eaten if one has problems of inflammation of ligaments, tendons and joints. For example, diabetic patients heal very badly and they are more prone to aches and pains, arthritis etc.

Posture

The secret of maintaining a healthy spine is to be constantly aware of your posture in wakefulness and sleep. Fatigue is one of the factors that contribute to bad posture and so exercises and sound sleep play an important role in the maintenance of its well-being.

It is advisable to seek the advice of an Alexander Technique or Pilates therapist to learn methods of maintaining good posture. Regular yoga also helps in this area.

At night it is important to choose the correct size of pillow. Ideally one should use a pillow that would fill in the gap between the neck and shoulder. If one prefers or habitually sleeps on the back, one should use a thinner pillow.

Massage

While having a shower or bath use a little soap (as a lubricant) and massage the muscles of the back of the neck and behind the ears. Use the forefingers and the thumb to rub the muscles and tendons, starting from the area where they are attached to the occiput (base of the skull) and going down to the base of the neck. While massaging one can expect to find one or more muscles to be quite painful and it is these tender muscles that need most attention.

If possible husbands and wives or partners should give each other a neck and shoulder massage for five minutes or so at bedtime. There is no better treatment for muscles than massage. Not only is it a direct hands-on treatment but it also gives comfort and relaxes the entire body. When you have a backache the muscles tense up, either due to the compression of the nerves in the affected segment of the spine or due to accumulation of lactic acid. Massage brings in more blood and therefore more oxygen, thus causing oxidation of the lactic acid to the end products (carbon dioxide and water).

This accumulation of lactic acid causes spasms of muscles and forms hardened 'knots' in them. They can be easily identified in the spinal muscles. These 'knots' interfere with the transmission of power along muscles by causing interruption in the pathway of muscles. They make muscles inert or less effective. Moreover these knots are sites of great pain and discomfort. If they are not released, then fibrous tissue may grow into them to immobilise them and make them inert. This is just a reaction of the body to isolate the problem. The hardened or fibrosed knots are a permanent site of pain in the spine. This condition is often referred to as fibromyalgia (fibro – fibrous tissue; myalgia – pain in muscles or myos).

The sooner these knots are flattened out in the muscles through massage, the better it is for the spine.

Technique

Use Dr Ali's Back Oil for massage. This oil consists of the following ingredients:

2 parts mustard oil

to warm the muscles and improve blood flow

½ part wintergreen oil

to soothe the muscles

½ part clove oil

as painkiller

4 parts sesame oil

to nourish (rich in vitamin E)

1 part black cumin seed oil

as anti-inflammatory remedy

The oil is massaged into the spinal muscles, which are easily identified along the length of the spine. It is important to massage along the entire spine, not just where the pain is, as the spinal muscles, not all of which run along the entire length of the spine, act as one. Together they create the anti-gravitational force. Rubbing only the sore areas will remove the immediate pain from it but will not help to treat the compression of discs, the root problem causing such pain.

Those who travel frequently, play strenuous and vigorous games, use computers a lot, drive for long hours or are stressed should seek professional help for their neck management. It would be advisable to see someone trained in the Ali Technique or the Alexander Technique once or twice a month as a preventative and therapeutic measure. If there is not any such therapist available then a deep tissue massage of the neck and spine as I have just described is very useful.

Sauna, Jacuzzi, vibrational chairs or beds, electrical devices that vibrate inside the cushions etc also relieve tensions from the spine in general.

Exercise

I recommend a series of yogic exercises that is designed to de-stress the body, replenish the energy and remove fatigue from the muscles. These exercises undertaken regularly are the best measures one can take to keep the spine supple and to correct the various postural and exertional defects that one acquires during the course of work and play.

The following exercises, which can be completed in 10–15 minutes (highly recommended soon after waking up), can keep your back in condition far into old age:

On the floor, face down

Cobra (half)

- Put the elbows by your sides.
- Take a deep breath in and raise your head looking up.
- Hold your breath for five seconds and slowly come down, breathing out. The forehead should touch the floor.
- Repeat this five times.

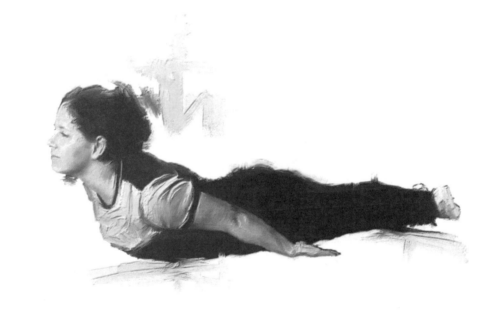

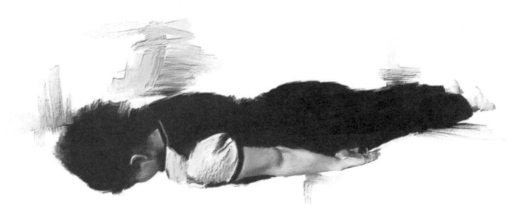

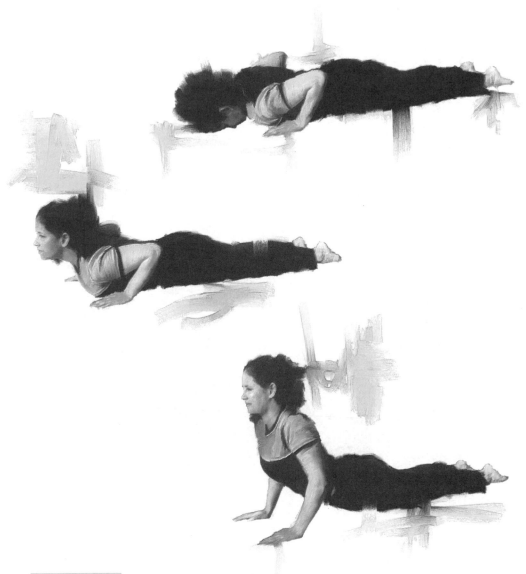

Cobra (full)

- Place your palms flat on the floor beside your shoulders.
- Take a deep breath in and lift your torso up and look up to the ceiling. The entire body is arched back with the help of the back muscles and the arms give it minimal support.
- Breathe out and gently return to the original position with forehead on the floor.
- Repeat this five times.

Modified swing

- Place both arms behind your back.
- Take a deep breath, hold the breath and lift your torso up, raising your head and feet above the floor. Look up as far as you can and stretch out, as if someone were pulling your feet away. The toes should be stretched outwards.
- Hold this position for five seconds and return to the original position, breathing out gently as you do so.
- Repeat this five times.

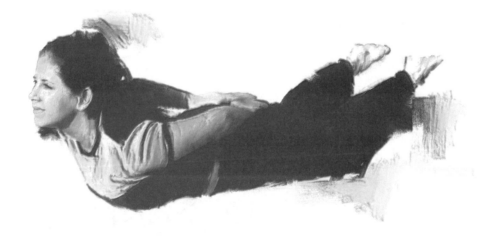

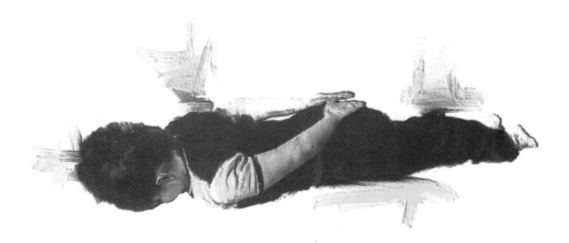

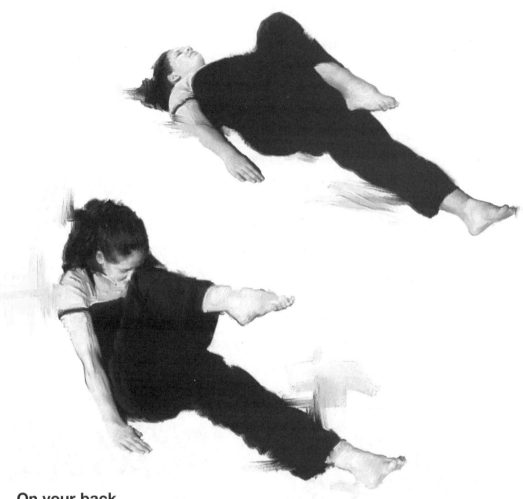

On your back

Child pose or pawan mukt

Sometimes called half-embryo or wind-releasing pose.

- Breathe in, bring your right knee to your chest, keep the left leg straight.
- Breathe out slowly, bringing your forehead to touch your knee.
- Lower your head to the floor slowly, keeping your chin towards your neck and breathing in.
- Breath out, relax arms and straighten leg.
- Repeat this with your other leg.
- Do this five times with each leg.

Spinal twist

- Extend arms at shoulder level.
- Bring knees up with feet on floor.
- Take a deep breath and turn your head to the left (ear should touch floor), while lowering your knees to the floor on the right (opposite direction).
- Breathe out and then breathe in and out very gently. As you do this you must make sure that your shoulders are flat on the floor. You should feel the twist in your spine and your knees will gradually descend to the floor as muscular tension is released from the lower back.
- Repeat the exercise turning your head to the right and letting your knees come down to the floor on the left.
- Repeat two or three times on each side.

This exercise will twist the spine to release spasm of muscles as well as help to align facet joints of vertebrae which get dislocated. This is a self-manipulative technique.

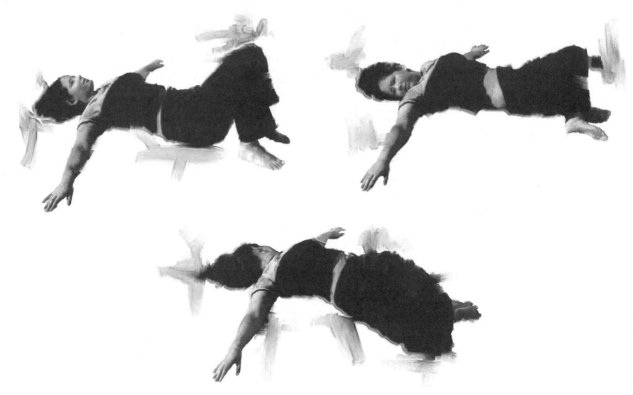

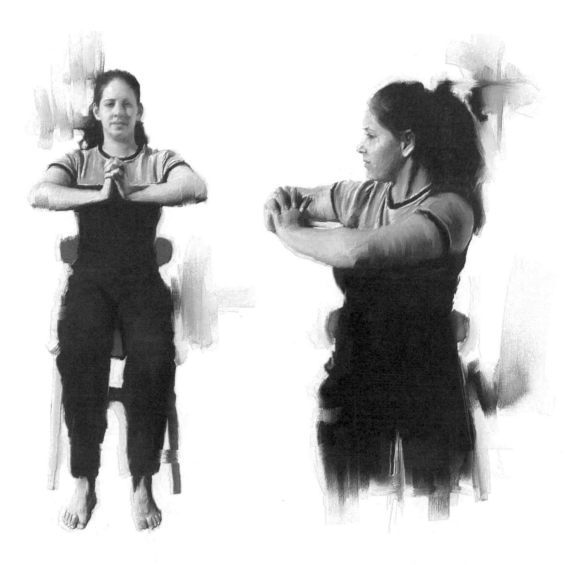

Sitting

Sitting spinal twist

- Sit upright on a chair or stool. Raise your elbows and clasp your hands in front of the chest.
- Breathe in as you twist to the right looking over your right shoulder. Breathe out slowly as you return to the original position.
- Do the same on the left.
- Do both five times.

Standing up

Arching back

- Stand with feet together. Tighten your seat (gluteal) muscles. Breathe in.
- Place both hands on the buttocks and push them forward. As you do this look up, arching your back. Do not bend your knees while doing this.
- Hold your breath for five seconds and return to the original position on breathing out.
- Repeat this five times. You should be able to feel the tension in your lower back and the release of it when you return to the original position.

This exercise will strengthen gluteal muscles and the lumbar muscles.

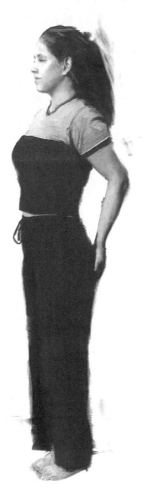 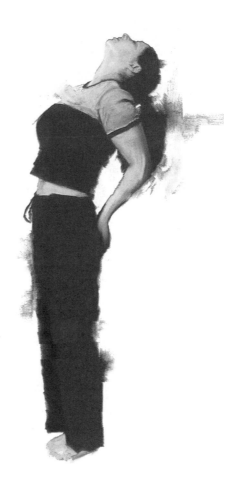

Neck twist

- Look ahead and grip your right shoulder (in the middle, not at the extremity) with the left hand. Place the right arm behind your back.
- Take a deep breath in and rotate your head towards the right, while simultaneously pulling the right shoulder forward with the left-hand. Hold your breath for five seconds. By doing this you will feel the stretch in the muscles of the right side of your neck and a release of tension in its joints.
- Return to the original position.
- Repeat the same with the other side.
- Do this five times in each direction.

This exercise will strengthen the muscles of the neck, improve movement of the neck in both directions, releasing the stiffness and shifting vertebrae that are out of alignment back into their original positions. This often acts like a self-manipulation.

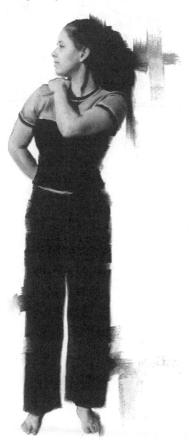

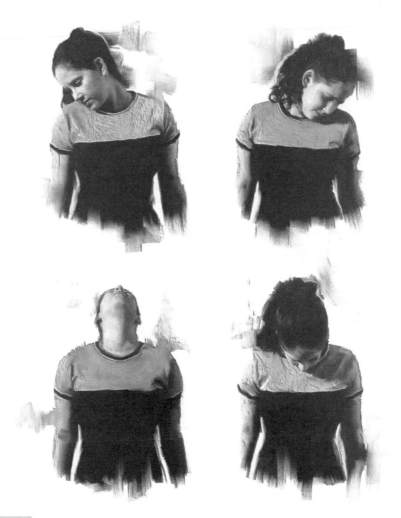

Head roll

- Bend your head so that the chin touches your chest.
- Rotate the head in a clockwise direction, making sure that parts of your head (chin, lower jaw, back of the head) touch your chest and shoulder throughout its journey. This way a total head roll is performed and the chances of dizziness are minimised.
- Do this five times and repeat in the anticlockwise direction.

This exercise will help to grind osteophytes or calcium deposits that so often settle on the joint surfaces all around. This releases the joints from stiffness.

Finally, lie on the floor face down for five minutes.

After being thoroughly loosened up try:

Self-traction

- Bend the arms at the elbows and join the palms of your hands to form a bowl. Rest your chin on this 'bowl' and place your palms on either side of your face. Your chin should rest firmly on the base of your palms.
- Join your elbows together, push them slightly forward and start to look up, so that you feel a traction in the neck. Breathe in and out very gently. On doing this, a stretch should be felt in your entire spine. Hold this position for a couple of minutes.

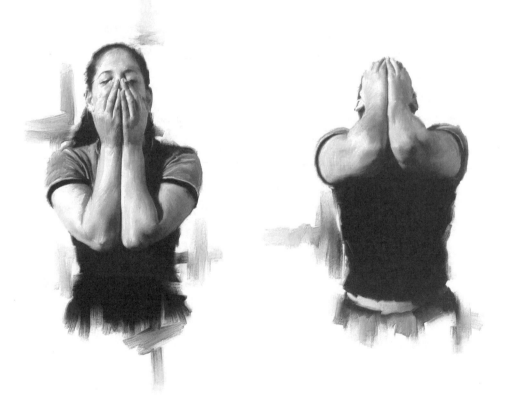

The above exercises are designed to work on muscles, tendons and joints. Thus they work on all parts that are directly involved in backache. They are good for both treatment and prevention of backache. But be careful not to stretch too far when you first start doing them. Build up slowly.

Deep Relaxation

Shavasana or Dead man's pose

One last exercise, which is very beneficial in cases of severe stress or backache, takes rather longer, so cannot be included in a normal quick workout. Regular use is recommended. To start with you may like to record the instructions below, at an appropriate slow pace, and play them back to remind you of the thoughts, but soon you will remember them. During this exercise your blood pressure may drop and you might feel slightly light-headed and a little cold due to the drop in the metabolic rate. Use a sheet to cover yourself while you do this exercise. Make sure that the door of your room is locked and the telephones are switched off. No one should disturb you while you do this. It is your 'prayer time', meant for your own relaxation and enlightenment.

- Lie on your back in a quiet place where you will not be disturbed. Make sure your clothes are loose, close your eyes, put your arms to your sides and relax. Loosen up all the joints – shoulders, elbows, wrists, fingers, knees, ankles and toes – by gently moving them.

- Take a deep breath in, counting three (approximately three seconds), pause for three seconds and breathe out very gently for six seconds. Initially it will be difficult to maintain this rhythm of breathing and you may find yourself out of breath. If you persevere you will be able to acquire that rhythm. When you breathe in let the belly blow out and when you breathe out let the abdominal wall cave in, pushing the diaphragm out. For the first couple of days just practise the breathing technique until everything is smooth. The ratio between inhalation and exhalation times should be 1:2.

- When you have acquired the correct breathing pattern, try concentration. Concentrate on your forehead, on the spot between your eyebrows. Imagine that you are looking at an orange spot, the rising or sinking sun. Feel the warmth on your forehead. Divert this warmth to the top and back of your skull and then to the sides and the temples. Imagine your brain relaxing and feeling warm. You can feel the thoughts, aches, pains, worries and stress simply evaporate. You feel your eyebrows relaxing and feeling warm. Next your eyelids feel light and relaxed. Your facial muscles and jaw muscles relax and feel warm.

- The back of your head feels warm and relaxed. Now your neck muscles feel warm and relaxed. Now your upper back feels warm and relaxed. Now your mid back feels warm and relaxed. Now your lower back feels warm and relaxed. Then your seat muscles, your thighs, your calves, your ankles and feet are relaxed. Experience the flow of warmth through these parts. You feel a gentle tingling sensation in your toes.

- Focus your attention again to the back of your head. Let the neck muscles feel warm and relaxed. This time let this sensation spread to the shoulders, the arms, elbows, forearms, wrists and to the tips of your fingers. You feel a little tingling in the tips of the fingers.

- Repeat the whole process a few times, concentrating on the trunk and legs, shoulders and arms, till your entire body feels calm and relaxed. You feel light and almost weightless.

- Concentrate on your heart and imagine that it is slowing down. Imagine that all the blood vessels are dilating and your blood pressure is dropping. Your body should feel totally relaxed. You may by now be in a state of trance – neither awake nor asleep.

- When you have enjoyed this state of relaxation, return to your wakeful situation. Breathe in, pushing your abdomen out and breathe out, taking your abdomen in. Do this in the same rhythmic pattern as when you started. After a few repeats of this, gently open your eyes and absorb the sights and sounds of the world very calmly.

- After this exercise do not do anything excitable and remain calm for a while. The exercise should last for 15–20 minutes. Do not count time, just train your mind to do this for the set time.

Philosophy of Exercises Involving the Mind

There is a constant theme running through the philosophies of the major exercise routines of the world, typically yoga, Bates Method exercises for the eyes, the Alexander Technique, Pilates, walking on uneven surfaces etc. They all build on the reconstitution of the control channels between brain and muscles in order to eliminate bad habits. In Hatha yoga, breathing is linked to physical movements so as to involve the subconscious brain. This alerts the brain to the ideal postures adopted and makes those patterns part of everyday habits.

In Bates Method eye exercises the distortion caused by bad habits is removed from the control channels to the brain so that fuzziness is replaced by sharp focus. Ask any person practising those routines, especially those who took them up in later life, and most will describe a short delay at their habitually worst focal length in attaining sharpness, suggesting that the bad habits are still remembered, but discarded by the brain in favour of better habits after the short delay.

Both Alexander and Pilates advocate overcoming bad habits in posture. Alexander in particular highlights the phenomenon that when students of the technique are asked to adopt a perfect posture they usually do not, yet think they have. Both techniques are devoted to teaching the student what good posture feels like and recording that in the subconscious brain in preference to the bad habit.

Walking on an uneven surface is actually following the same philosophy, by activating the reflexes to react accurately to the stimulus of unexpected placement of the feet. At first you stagger and lose balance because your brain has been lulled into inertia and laziness by a sedentary or repetitive lifestyle, but soon the accurate balance returns and allows you to skip from rock to rock in confidence and perfect balance. The posture-maintaining muscles have been toned up and incidentally the pressure on the discs has been relieved.

What should be a matter of concern to everyone is that mindless aerobic exercise does not address this need. The person who walks for an hour on a walking machine, maybe watching the TV, has done nothing to overcome the bad habits of his posture-maintaining muscles. Jogging on a treadmill for a mile and thinking of problems, listening to music or the radio, or even thinking of nothing, may do plenty for your circulatory system but does little for your posture-maintaining muscles or your bad habits, and may even damage your spine if you run with even a vestige of a stoop. Weightlifting is a particularly repetitive exercise which may do more harm than good if it unbalances the development and toning of superficial muscles at the expense of those maintaining posture.

I believe these mindless aerobic exercises were an outcome of people's desire to work hard and work out hard. Perhaps they were developed by people with an obsessive behavioral pattern that just wanted to do repetitive things, like a child spinning round and round in a Hula-Hoop or skipping, simply to get rid of surplus energy. From teenage days people do push-ups, use rowing machines and do all these monotonous work-outs. Unfortunately, if you are in this sort of hyped-up situation throughout the day or under stress, you do not want extra adrenalin to be generated. By joining the constant quest for more and more whoomf, you ultimately end up in a state where your heart is better, you can justify the excess butter and cheese that you have consumed during the day, you have been able to oxygenate your body much better, but ultimately your mind will be neglected and it will be in that constant state of alertness which society and industry want us to achieve all the time.

The sensible thing to do is the exact opposite. The antidote is to do slow and calming exercises, so that you breathe, as you do in Alexander Technique, tai chi, yoga and Pilates, all correcting techniques which teach you to maintain good posture. Also Alexander Technique and Pilates both require that you have a teacher. If you do these exercises well, they will produce those chemicals and hormones in the body which have a very calming effect. The balance between excitement and calmness is very essential in one's life. You cannot be in a heightened state from the morning all the way through the day – get up at five, go to work, rush around and maybe dance till late in the evening. At weekends, you crash out. After all that, today's young people are exhausted. They work so hard, even the food is delivered to them at their desk.

The result is that they squander their youthful energy. 21-year-olds, particularly, get drawn into this turmoil. They continue reckless exploitation of their bodies until, by the time they are 25 or 26, they catch the most horrendous colds and infections. It pulls down the immune system. A lot of them crack up.

If they do exercises and take a lot of vitamins and pills, these may mask the damage, which becomes less apparent but is still there. They take drinks that dilate blood vessels, with caffeine and other chemicals, so they artificially maintain their energy, obviously aging their body to the limit. Unless you slow down your mechanism the body is going to age. The faster the pace of life, the more activities you do, the faster your body clock runs. If you sleep four hours a night, night after night, and take medicines to keep you going, you keep leaping forward in effective age. If you are supposed to work for eight hours, but you work for 16, it means you work for two days in the span of one day and the same things happen. That's how the body will interpret it. Two days in 24 hours. There are, of course, exceptions such as Winston Churchill, born with an exceptional constitution, who lived to a great age yet lived like that, but these are exceptions. Here we are discussing the general population. The body does not like continuous generation of energy. If you put a sentry outside to guard the barracks, he has to sit down somewhere after four hours to recover. Otherwise he will report sick.

When flying in aircraft the same thing applies. If there is high risk or danger (one is increasingly aware of this now since 11 September 2001) then the journey becomes very stressful and draining, which can be extremely harmful to one's health. There are rules. In Russia this control of energy is practiced extensively. For example Russian miners have four months of holiday per year. Schoolteachers the world over are given long holidays because the stress of looking after young children is very great. For the same reason school terms are becoming shorter and shorter because of the high pressure. Boarding schools have longer holidays than day schools. School authorities say it is to give the children more time with their parents. In fact it is for the teachers, who are under enormous stress 24 hours a day.

Sleep

As mentioned earlier, sleep is very important for muscles as it is in a deep and comfortable sleep that the muscles and ligaments get an opportunity to rest and replenish the lost energy. In wakefulness or disturbed sleep, the muscles are in a tonic state (tensed) while in deep sleep they are completely relaxed. The spine can comfortably take a few hours (four to six) of supporting itself in a vertical position at a time. The neck muscles in the waking state continuously support the heavy head throughout the day. A short nap or siesta after lunch is highly recommended to give the neck a rest.

One should avoid eating late in the evening as the process of digestion (movement of the intestines, release of gas, heavy food) can disturb sleep. Disturbing films or newscasts that focus on violence on television often cause excitement in the mind and affect the quality of sleep. One should read something pleasant or listen to soothing music before going to bed. Sleep is also disturbed by dehydration at night. It is best to drink some water before going to sleep and use the toilet to empty the bladder, as rising to do so is another disturbing factor at night.

Sarangi, an ancient Indian musical instrument, produces in my opinion the right vibrational sound to soothe the mind. It makes a sound that is almost identical to a soothing human voice. In India a 'Lori' or bedtime lullaby has a most powerful hypnotic effect on a child before it is put to sleep. It resonates in the mind and relaxes the muscles to a state where sleep is imminent.

Ustad Sultan Khan, one of the greatest exponents of the Sarangi and a phenomenal singer of devotional songs (Sufi songs dedicated to the Almighty), has created a few Loris or lullaby songs which he has sung, as well as played on his instrument, for my therapeutic use. I recommend this music be played at bedtime as it produces the vibrations in the mind that induce sleep. This soothing music relaxes muscles, slows down the heart rate and prepares the body for sleep. It breaks the barrier of language as it consists of human voice and sounds of nature, which are universal.

It is no wonder that Lord Yehudi Menuhin, having heard this music, said 'Sarangi is the music of the soul'. People have been known to become emotional and often weep with joy during live performances with this instrument.

Finally, always remember, a healthy spine supports a healthy mind.

Chapter 9

Carrying Out an MOT

So far in this book we have studied how the back works, how to take care of it, service it and maintain it. There is one other operation necessary to keep any machine in good order and that is to periodically test it for symptoms that might lead to trouble. In the case of my own body or spine I call this My Own Testing, or MOT, just like the people who test your car. It is an important tool and from time to time you must do an assessment of your back. We know how important it is to check our car – how much more so our own backs!

Backache depends on a few major factors, the amount of **weight** you carry, the amount of **stress** you have, your personal **nutritional** state, your **posture** and your **exercise** plan. These are the five different factors that we need to identify.

Weight

In the weight category, you need to ask yourself the question: are you carrying excess weight, are you obese? Excess weight puts stress on the lower back, the joints, the discs and the heart. It is also an indicator of plaque formation in the arteries and joints, lack of exercise, indulgence and ill-health. If you have excess weight the heart has to work that much harder to supply oxygen and you need more energy to carry yourself around. If you are not doing exercises the muscles are not fit enough and the pressure on the discs of the spine increases. The anti-gravitational force provided by the intervertebral muscles is overwhelmed. You are at risk of disc compressions and injuries to the hip and knee joints. It could be a continuous strain on your body.

You need to know three things about your weight:

- What is your optimum weight?
- What is your normal weight?
- How much has it changed recently?

It is very important to try and maintain your optimum weight.

There is a quick rule of thumb to calculate your optimum weight. Subtract 100 from your height in centimetres and that is your ideal weight in kilograms. (If the height is 160 cm and you take away 100, it gives you an ideal weight of 60 kgs; if your height is 180 cm your ideal weight would be 80 kgs).

The next step is to find your normal weight; just take an average over the past few weighings. If there is a significant difference between your normal weight and what it should be you need to so something about it. But remember, there can be individual variations. A muscular person's ideal weight could be above the average; that of a woman with osteoporosis might be below average. Furthermore, if you take a lot of exercise much of any 'excess' weight could be muscle and that is perfectly healthy.

If you are doing regular exercises, you may be able to cope with some excess weight (within reason) without back tension, breathlessness when you walk upstairs or lethargy (especially in the early morning when you feel sluggish). If all these physical signs are OK your weight is OK. A 10 per cent increase on your ideal weight, however, is the danger limit. (So for a person of 80 kgs, then 88 kgs is the danger limit.) That's when the body will start to act up, especially the lower back – one of the commonest sites for weight-related problems.

Finally, if your recent weighings show an upward trend, then you must take action. Sometimes, however, women over the age of 50 or 60, after losing weight (due to calcium loss in the bones), start putting it on again, only because they are gaining muscle and depositing calcium in the bones, especially if they exercise regularly. Weight loss is often through expulsion of water that we tend to retain. When I put people on healthy diets they lose weight quite rapidly in the first month or so. Then they plateau. The waist measurement may still reduce but not the weight. This is because the diet is combined with exercise, which creates muscle mass, and this weighs more than fat.

If you want to work out your ideal weight more scientifically, then follow the World Health Organisation (WHO) guidelines. According to WHO, obesity is defined as a condition in which there is an excess of body fat. Body Mass Index (BMI), a calculation of build, is used to indicate the level of obesity. To work out your BMI: divide your weight (in kilograms) by the square of your height (in metres).

Metric weight (kg) ÷ height (m)

or:

Imperial weight (lbs) x 704 ÷ height (ins)

A normal BMI is in the range 18.5–24.9

You are overweight if your BMI is in the range 25.0–29.9

You are obese if your BMI is more than 30

WHO advises that generally, as a person's BMI increases, the risk of disease and other obesity-related conditions, particularly back problems, rises too. (Interestingly, in Asia, the onset of these conditions occurs on average at a lower BMI, to such an extent that Regional Obesity Guidelines have had to be issued. An example of individuality ignored by the statisticians until recently.)

Whichever method you use you should now be able to compare your ideal weight with what it is and take action to correct it if necessary.

Stress

Next the stress level. Here you have to ask yourself basically the following questions:

● do you sleep well or not? If you do not sleep regularly or sleep well, say less than three nights per week, then the muscles will not be in a state of relaxation. If you sleep well for less than three nights a week then it is pretty sure you will suffer from some sort of backache, especially neck ache.

- are you so stressed as to get neck ache and muscle ache? This should be classified as moderate to severe.
- do you travel a lot, especially across time zones? This adds to the stress.
- do you have any ongoing illnesses in your body? Do these worry you?
- do you have personal or financial problems, are they worries? This includes deadlines and dilemmas.
- do you drink a lot of coffee, and other stimulants that can stress you?

Diet

Next the nutritional aspect. Ask yourself the following questions:

- are you drinking too much acid, for example orange juice? Too much acid will cause inflammation of the ligaments and tendons, and may cause interference in the weight-bearing capacity.
- do you take excess alcohol or drinks containing caffeine? These can also dehydrate muscles in the long run, which can interfere with the transmission of power.
- how much water do you drink? If you drink too little water then the kidney area in the lumbar region will be very sore and that can interfere with the transmission of muscle power and cause weakness in the lower back.
- do you take excess salt? If you take too much salt then the muscles will be tight and tensed.
- do you take recreational drugs, which interfere with your state of alertness such as marijuana, cocaine and other relaxants. I also include in this category medicinal/nutritional supplements/drugs, tranquillisers, sedatives and anxiety pills such as St John's wort, Valeriana, Kava kava etc. They tend to de-power your muscles, which can cause problems. Do you take aspirin, contraceptive pills, hormone replacement drugs or excessive antibiotics? These can also interfere with muscles and can cause excessive bruising and sluggishness.

- do you smoke? Nicotine can cause a slowdown of the flow of blood in the muscles.
- are you a strict vegetarian? If so you are highly likely to have calcium deficiencies which can cause muscular cramps. Calcium deficiencies may cause degeneration or bone loss and eventually degeneration in the bones and in the joints.

Posture

Posture and other related problems lead to the following questions:

- are you in a profession where you are continuously lifting and carrying? What do you do to manage that, to counteract the effects?
- are you sitting in front of computers for more than two hours at a time without a break? Or up to eight hours a day? This will definitely produce neck tension.
- are you leaning over a desk all the time?
- are you driving? How much do you drive? If you drive in excess of 15 hours a week then you are in trouble.
- How much flying are you doing? Flying always dehydrates and causes postural problems, especially if you are always travelling in economy class.

Lifestyle

We have covered weight, posture, sleep, stress, so we have to ask questions about lifestyle:

- do you get up fresh in the morning or do you suffer early morning stiffness in the back or in the joints?
- at the end of the day do you feel so tired as to go and slump into a chair or do you feel fine?
- how much exercise do you do? Moderate, or none?
- do you do weightlifting, how much of it? Fitness has nothing to do with backache. Do you do certain injurious sports like squash (they very often

injure the gluteal regions) or high-impact aerobics? Then you need to take care.

Self-diagnosis of the Back

Besides carrying out the above tests to identify any signs of forthcoming backache, there are direct and indirect ways of finding out whether you might have problems.

1

Lie down on the carpet, relax your heels, your knees, your hips and your shoulders. Wriggle about to find a comfortable position. Then breathe in and out. If you get any tension in the lower back, mid back or upper back, as the muscles relax and the spine is stretched, you know there are some problems in the associated area.

2

Being in this position, rotate your back to the left, pointing your nose towards your left shoulder, and see how far you can go. If you cannot reach the maximum rotated position, when the ear lobes touch the floor, if there are restrictions of pain, you know that there are some problems either in the joints, facet joints, on the left side of the cervical spine or that there are excited muscles or ligaments in the opposite side, the right side, which are preventing this movement. Then you do the same on the other side.

3

Gently lift your neck and bring the chin closer to the chest. If there is any pain, then you know there are some problems here too. Try to identify the area that hurts most.

4

Bend your knees, draw your ankles closer to your hips. Keep the feet apart to the width of the hips. Look straight up and let the knees drop to one side and gently breathe in and out and see how far they go. If the lower knee does not touch the floor – normally it should go right down to the floor – then there are certain problems in your lumbar spine. Try to identify the area that hurts. Do the same on the opposite side.

5

Lie flat with the legs stretched, lift your right leg up and keep the knees straight. Lift it right up and see how far it goes. If it reaches 90 degrees (straight up) then your hips and lower back are fine. If it does not then there are certain muscular spasms preventing it from doing so. Do the same with the left leg.

6

Stand up straight, with your arms ahead of you and try to touch your toes with knees straight to see if you can go down to about 60 degrees. Within five inches of your toes or nearer is fine. If you cannot bend that far then something is wrong.

7

Stand up, clasp your hands in front of your chest and rotate your spine from your hips, keeping the pelvis straight. If you twist less than 90 degrees, identify the area that hurts.

8

Still standing, rotate the neck gently around the axis in both directions. If there are crackling noises they need to be freed up. If there is any dizziness then there are some problems. There should be no crackling noises and no dizziness.

9

Stand up and cough a few times. If there is any pain in any of the areas of the spine then that area needs attention. If there is no pain then your discs are likely to be fine.

Age

Between 60 and 70, when growth retards, there is the possibility of some age-related wear and tear. These are called the osteoarthritic changes. This is a natural process, because Nature does not expect you to go on for ever and ever with the lissomness of youth. It is a way of slowing down. It's a caution. So certain ligaments calcify, and then they restrict your movements. But if you practise the yoga exercises in Chapter 8, such exercises twist and turn every aspect of the body. Then your back can be kept supple. You will find you can do a bit more than if you aged normally, because you have listened to the Messages of Nature. Then the body feels that you need not restrict yourself and lets you go on.

Questionnaire

Many people and companies believe in an annual checkup. In the majority of cases, however, such tests fail to show our state of health. They only show whether infections are present and whether the body constants, the homeostasis, are right or not – blood pressure, blood count, cholesterol level, heart function and so on. Because our bodies have a phenomenal capacity to keep these constants in balance within ourselves, very rarely do these parameters change. Some companies send their executives to very expensive clinics, spending up to US$50,000 on each, and the limited relevance of the results is hardly cost-effective. Such tests confirm the client is free from disease, but tells you very little about his state of health, in particular almost nothing about the state of his back. Almost never are you tested for the condition of your back.

You can, however, find out all you need to know about the health of your back – for nothing. Give some thought to the five factors I have discussed above, go through the nine diagnostic tests, then answer the MOT questionnaire. Do it privately and honestly, to yourself. Don't think too much about the questions, as you should have done all the necessary thinking by now. Just answer quickly and firmly. The result should tell you if your back is in great shape, whether it needs some tuning up you can do yourself, or whether you need help.

My Own Testing for the Back

Tick the appropriate box

Physical

		Normal/Yes	Nearly	Abnormal/No
1	Weight	❏	❏	❏
2	Supine, breathe deeply in and out. Pain?	❏	❏	❏
3	Supine, can touch floor with ear? Pain?	❏	❏	❏
4	Supine, chin to chest – pain?	❏	❏	❏
5	Supine, knees bent, twist touch floor each side?	❏	❏	❏
6	Supine, lift each leg up to vertical?	❏	❏	❏
7	Stand, can touch toes?	❏	❏	❏
8	Stand, arms out, twist to 90 degrees?	❏	❏	❏
9	Stand, rotate neck. Cracking noises or dizziness? Chin can touch shoulder?	❏	❏	❏
10	Stand up and cough. Any pain in spine?	❏	❏	❏
11	Stand up and arch backwards. Pain?	❏	❏	❏
12	Sleep with less than two pillows?	❏	❏	❏
13	Back stiffness and pain on getting up?	❏	❏	❏

Stress

		Seldom	Sometimes	Frequently
1	Excessively tired?	❏	❏	❏
2	Sleep badly?	❏	❏	❏
3	Dilemmas and deadlines?	❏	❏	❏
4	Travel long distances?	❏	❏	❏
5	Rely on stimulants?	❏	❏	❏
6	Headaches?	❏	❏	❏
7	Anxiety/panic attacks?	❏	❏	❏

Nutritional

		Seldom	Sometimes	Frequently
1	Stomach acid-making foods?	❑	❑	❑
2	Too little water? (should be 6–8 glasses a day)	❑	❑	❑
3	Too few vegetables?	❑	❑	❑
4	Not enough calcium + vitamin D?	❑	❑	❑
5	Too much chocolate, wine, bread, coffee?	❑	❑	❑
6	Take recreational drugs?	❑	❑	❑
7	Take prescribed drugs, tranquillisers, sedatives?	❑	❑	❑

Posture

		Seldom	Sometimes	Frequently
1	Suffer backache?	❑	❑	❑
2	Suffer neckache?	❑	❑	❑
3	Work with computers?	❑	❑	❑
4	Heavy lifting?	❑	❑	❑
5	Lean over? (e.g. desk, artist's easel)	❑	❑	❑
6	Drive long distances?	❑	❑	❑
7	Sit badly? (home, work, aeroplane)	❑	❑	❑

Lifestyle

		Seldom	Sometimes	Frequently
1	Potentially injurious exercise?	❑	❑	❑
2	Not enough calming exercises? (yoga, tai chi, Alexander, Pilates, walking)	❑	❑	❑
3	Mindless exercises? (aerobics, jogging)	❑	❑	❑
4	Morning stiffness?	❑	❑	❑
5	Not enough massage?	❑	❑	❑
6	Rely on supplements?	❑	❑	❑

Ali Syndrome (constriction of vertebral arteries in the neck, through disalignment)

	Seldom	Sometimes	Frequently
1 Blurrred vision, dizziness, nausea, tinnitus, hyperventilation and palpitation, chronic fatigue?	❏	❏	❏
2 Short-term memory loss, confusion and lack of verbal expression, stuttering?	❏	❏	❏
3 Autoimmune disorders, poor immune system with frequent coughs and colds, allergies?	❏	❏	❏
4 Loss of libido, menstrual dysfunctions in women, impotence?	❏	❏	❏
5 Depression, disturbed sleep, mood swings, craving for sugar, burning mouth syndrome?	❏	❏	❏

	A	B	C
Total			

Calculate 2 x A + B = [   ]

60 or more your back is OK

70 or more your back is excellent

80 or more your back is outstanding

90 either you are very young, an Olympic gymnast or you cheated.

Less than 50 you should seriously consider changes in your lifestyle.

Less than 40 you should visit an integrated medical doctor, chiropractor or osteopath. If the low marks were derived from bad posture join a yoga, Alexander or Pilates class.

PART II

WHEN THINGS GO WRONG

Chapter **10**

Genesis of Backache

Before we look at the origin of backache we must look into the development of the spine from the foetal stage. In the initial stage the bones have no role to play and therefore all the body's energy is spent in developing organs and systems that are vital. Circulation is the most important parameter of life. If there is no heartbeat one is pronounced dead. The circulatory system provides nutrition and removes toxins or waste products. Thus its development takes priority.

During the entire process of development in the womb, the bones grow as the muscles grow. The foetus floats in the womb, swims, kicks and often does somersaults. These movements bring joy to the mother as they are the first sign of life that the unborn demonstrates. All the bones connected with leg and arm movements develop simultaneously with the spinal bones.

As the baby is born, the risk of damage to the spine is high, especially if it is an abnormal birth. A rapid or lightning-like birth can cause just as much damage as a slow and tedious birth. The quick movement through the birth canal may twist and turn the baby in different directions in a short period of time. A slow and tedious birth produces trauma to the spine as it is twisted and turned several times during numerous powerful contractions of the uterus. The neck, being the most fragile part of the spine, and since most babies are born head-first, is frequently traumatised at birth. If the head is blocked by one of the bony structures of the pelvis then contractions may cause compressions of the neck. These traumas range from dislocation of vertebrae and stretched ligaments to compressed discs. It is not until years later that these damaged parts show signs of pathology or discomfort.

In breach position, the baby goes through a very difficult situation as the buttocks are 'docked' into the birth canal. The hip is wider than the width of the skull and unless the size of the baby is really small or the birth canal large, labour in this position is always very strenuous and difficult. Ultimately, there is only one solution, namely to tilt the hip to one side so that it enters the birth canal in an oblique position and inches through it very slowly. This tilting of the hip results in shifting of its delicate joints and bony structures. This may result in a semi-permanent tilting of the hip which is one of the main reasons for scoliosis and shortening of one of the legs. Injuries to the gluteal muscles may lead to spasms in later years, causing sciatica. These injuries show signs of pathology years later. There is always an 'inborn' spinal defect when babies are born in breach positions. Traditional Indian midwives take breach positions very seriously and they do their best to reverse the positions in the womb, before birth, by using manipulative art and massage. Babies born in breach positions are said to grow up to have lower back pain and sciatica in later years. There is also a very interesting saying in folk remedies in India (probably circulated by the Dais): 'If you have low backache, go and ask a man born in the breach position to massage the back with his left foot and it will get cured.' Why a man born in breach position and why the left foot will remain a mystery. I suspect that when dealing with breach positions, the experienced midwives try to pull the baby down with the right hip first and therefore the left leg is stronger or less traumatised as one presumes that the left leg is innately weak and one does not want to weaken it any further by causing further damage. Only statistics can prove this.

If you look at the skull and face of newborn babies the deformations on them will tell you what pressure they must have endured during birth. Thankfully, the skull bones are not joined together at birth and the fontanelles are there, otherwise the skull would be crushed like an eggshell.

Newborn babies lie on their back most of the time. They kick around, strengthening their limb muscles, which in a few weeks become strong enough to grasp, and push with their legs. Back muscles however develop more slowly. The baby begins to raise the head at about four months but it can move the head from side to side, for example to follow an object with its eyes, even earlier. The head is fairly heavy and therefore it is a while before the baby can lift it but it is able to hold its neck in the vertical position by two months of age. As it grows it begins to hold its back upright and at about five to six months it can sit up supporting the spine vertically. At this point mechanical traumas are the only risk to the spine. As soon as the child begins to stand and then walk at the end of the first year, the chances of traumas to the spine increase as it frequently falls when learning to move.

Usually the first sign of backache starts at teenage. It is often termed as 'growing pains'. The bones grow very fast – at a phenomenal rate. In fact teenagers are growing much faster these days, probably caused by their eating habits; I suspect antibiotic- or hormone-treated meats could be the cause. Stress may be stimulating the growth hormone in the pituitary gland. This acceleration in height, sometimes several inches in a year, causes many problems to the body. The rapid bone growth is not compensated by equally quick development of muscles. The muscles can't keep pace with the growth of the bones and therefore get stretched. Injuries take place in the tendons or muscles at both ends where maximum stretching or tension is experienced. That is why in 'growing pains' the tendons of the spinal muscles in the occiput or nape of the neck and lower back (near the sacrum) hurt most. Pains are also experienced above the knee, around the tendons of the quadriceps. The growth of the bone leads to stretching of tendons like the strings of a bow that is being pulled straight. The tightness of muscles and ligaments of the spine, in some cases, may cause the discs of the vertebral column, especially the lumbar and cervical regions, to get compressed. This can cause serious backache, which may be prolonged beyond the period when growth stops.

In an adult, backache is caused by the following structures:

Muscles, ligaments and tendons

The common source of backache is muscles. When muscles contract they need oxygen to convert glucose into energy. If they work very hard then the demand for oxygen grows but the supply is constant. Therefore some of the glucose gets partially burnt into lactic acid, instead of totally burning into carbon dioxide and water, as is the case when the oxygen supply is in abundance. If a person is up for long hours for several days at a stretch, the muscles become fatigued as more lactic acid accumulates in them. Lactic acid and calcium deficiency cause muscles to go into local spasm, also known as 'knots'. Lactic acid irritates nerve fibres and causes pain. A hot tub/bath or a good massage on the spine takes this sort of pain away quite quickly as the blood circulation improves and the lactic acid is oxidised to carbon dioxide and water. Stretching and exercises can also relieve this sort of backache as muscles get toned up and the supply of blood to them increases.

Physical work can also strain muscles, especially if heavy lifting or carrying is involved. Muscles can get inflamed and cause backache. Bad posture at work, or anywhere for that matter, is also a frequent cause of muscular backache. Sitting in one position for a long time causes the postural muscles to tire and this generates aches in them.

Tendons attached to muscles, in my experience, are the most common structures from where backache is generated. Strained muscles can repair themselves quite quickly as they have a rich network of blood vessels, but ligaments have very poor blood supply. That is why muscles are red or pink in colour while the tendons are white in colour. Only small blood vessels supply the tendons as they are tough and fibrous. The thick collagen fibres of tendons make them as tough as steel cords and suitable for attachment to bones and cartilages. Muscles are too soft to have direct attachment to bones and their fibres would tear with the slightest strain or stress. Nature therefore provided tendons at both ends of muscles to give them the extra strength to bear the force of contraction so that they can pull and facilitate movements at joints.

Tendons, when injured, take longer to heal because of the poor blood supply. Soft tissues like muscles heal quicker than tough or hard tissues like tendons, ligaments, bones and cartilages. Injured tendons become inflamed and they have:

a

swelling ('tumour' in Latin)

b

redness ('rubor')

c

pain ('bolor')

d

heat ('calor')

e

loss of function ('functio laesa')

f

hardness ('dolor').

Inflamed tendons have swelling, pain and loss of function. In the back these symptoms are manifested as backache, stiffness of the back (loss of movement or function) and swelling (can be felt palpatorily). Tendons thus are frequent causes of backache. Long working hours lead to straining of the tendons. Doing the same job (lifting, bending, carrying etc) over and over again leads to repetitive strain injuries (RSI) of the tendons of the back muscles. Sports injuries caused by sudden unplanned movements or falls strain the tendons of back muscles. Unless treated these strained and injured tendons can be inflamed for a long time. As they cannot be diagnosed by X-rays or scans, these injuries can remain undetected and yet continue to cause discomfort in the back. Anti-inflammatory drugs cannot reach the tendons, as the blood supply is poor, so painkillers are unfortunately the only option as they mask the pain for a few hours at a time. In my opinion, these tendon injuries are poorly diagnosed by physiotherapists and orthopaedic surgeons while most chronic backaches fall into this category of tendon-related back problems.

Loss of function of tendons weakens the anti-gravitational force that keeps the spine erect. This leads to the compression of the discs, especially between the lower (lumbar region) vertebrae where the weight of the torso and upper part of the body has to be borne. The compression of the discs leads to further complication of backaches as neurological symptoms develop (sciatica, foot drop etc). Thus disc problems are secondary in most cases, not primary as orthopaedics have led us to believe so far. In my experience, the problem first starts with the muscles and tendons before progressing into disc problems. Of course accidents, falls and other traumas can cause direct injury to the discs at the moment of impact, but these are relatively rare. Even then muscles act as shock absorbers protecting the discs. However, weak muscles reduce the shock-absorbing quality and high impact can overcome it.

Ligaments are fibrous sheaths that cover joint surfaces. They reinforce the joints so that the two bones that form them are tightly bound and yet reasonably flexible to allow movement in them. Joints, like hinges, must move and yet they must be stable to allow very little scope for dislocation. If they were not adequately fixed the two surfaces of the joints would slip out or dislocate. Ligaments facilitate this fixture of joint surfaces. Strain, stress and injuries weaken these ligaments. Constant stretching in awkward directions, as at work or during sports, can make the ligaments around joints loose. This creates an ideal situation for joints to dislocate or slip out of their alignment. On their own, joints dislocate when there is a sudden torsion or a force that moves them unexpectedly. This happens during an accident or a fall. In this case there is a traumatic dislocation of joints. Ligaments when injured due to above-mentioned factors can be inflamed. This can cause chronic ache in parts of the back where these are damaged. Like tendons, ligaments too have very poor blood supply and are therefore white in colour. They heal badly with conventional methods of treatment and therefore become a constant source of pain.

Joints

Dislocation of joints in the spine leads to the disalignment of vertebrae. When that happens, the discs are squeezed inappropriately causing them to bulge and rupture, ultimately irritating nerve roots that emerge from the spinal cord laterally. A sudden bulge or rupture of a disc can irritate or compress the nerve roots, causing great pain. This is known as 'slipped disc', a misleading term as discs are too gelatinous to 'slip' and can only protrude or rupture. The result can also be referred pain to the groin, leg, buttocks etc (in the direction of the nerves). Manipulations of the vertebrae can reinstate the alignment. Joints of the spine can be inflamed due to wear and tear or rheumatic changes. This is when osteoarthritis or rheumatoid arthritis can set in. These arthritic changes can cause pain and stiffness in the back, especially in the morning.

Bones

Bone mass as such has no nerve endings and therefore cannot hurt or feel pain. Bones are hard, and soft nerves cannot penetrate them as they usually survive in delicate, blood-rich surroundings. Therefore if there is any pathology inside the bone, the body usually does not know about it. Thus a bone tumour is often not detected or is symptom-less, unless it is large enough to destroy the outer layer of the bones (known as periosteum; peri – surrounding as in 'perimeter', os – bone) where there are numerous nerve endings. Thus most bone-related pain in the backbone originates from the surface or joints of the vertebrae. Osteoporosis, tuberculosis, bone tumours and other pathologies of the bone, manifest themselves only when they have destroyed the vertebral bodies (bone mass) enough to reach the outer surfaces, when of course severe and continuous pain is felt. Fractures of parts of vertebrae are very painful as the outer surface is traumatised.

Discs

As mentioned earlier, discs are involved in the genesis of backache in a secondary way most of the time. Primary disc conditions arise out of acute trauma or injury, as in an accident or fall. Discs can degenerate due to age when the blood supply to them gets affected. If the person puts on a lot of weight, the pressure on the discs increases and after some time the sac that contains the gelatinous substance becomes weak in a certain area. This makes the disc bulge with the substance penetrating into the softened area. Just as a stretched balloon becomes easy to blow up, due to loss of elasticity, the discs too can bulge without offering resistance when their walls are stretched and weakened. Once a disc bulges for the first time, it creates a weakness in its walls. It can then bulge again and again in future. This explains why people get recurrent attacks of 'slipped disc' if they do not look after their spine. Therefore it is very important to take preventive measures like weight loss, exercises, nutrition etc to manage the spine after the first acute attack.

Sometimes discs rupture due to trauma or other factors that weaken their sacs over a long period of time. The ruptured disc can impinge the nerve and cause permanent backache with a range of neurological symptoms. A ruptured disc is difficult to manage conservatively and often requires surgical intervention. This is the worst type of back problem as the very integrity of an important structure of the back is affected.

With age the gelatinous substance in the discs loses moisture. This causes the discs to shrink and flatten, thus narrowing the gap between the vertebrae. As a result of this narrowing some nerve roots may be trapped (or facet joints can become out of line and unduly worn) and cause substantial pain in the back. That is why, in old age, people get backache quite frequently.

It must be noted that the vertebrae of the neck, being very mobile, are more prone to injuries. Thus the chance of neck pain occurring in the routine course of a lifetime is very high. The thoracic vertebrae are fixed with the ribs and the sternum and therefore do not move so easily. The thoracic spine is fixed to provide additional protection to the vital organs like the heart and the lungs. The lumbar spine is very prone to injuries as the vertebrae are not only relatively mobile (to facilitate twisting and turning) but are also empowered with the task of supporting the weight of the upper body.

Referred pain

There are a lot of referred pains from internal organs into the back. These include pain caused by kidneys, renal stones, colon problems, uterine problems etc. Inflammation, cancer and ulcerations in these organs can cause pain that is often referred to the lower back. Similarly gallstones, collapsed lungs, stomach ulcers, pancreatitis etc can cause referred pain in the upper or mid back. Sometimes dislocations of ribs at the point of attachment may cause severe mid-back pain. Shingles, a viral infection affecting nerves, can cause backache.

Examples of referred pain

Joseph, 50, was an American gentleman in a high-powered job, which had its own stresses. He was debilitated with a low backache for over four months. He tried chiropractic, acupuncture, physiotherapy, massage, stress management etc with temporary or no relief. The MRI scan showed a mild bulge of the lower lumbar discs and the surgeons were contemplating surgery.

He called me and I flew over to New York and saw him the same evening. I examined him thoroughly and it was clear that the main spasm was in the lower mid back. Moreover his pain did not radiate along the sciatic nerve, as the lower lumbar discs would have caused. His discs were clearly not the problem.

I inquired about his diet to evaluate his kidney problems because that is the area that was sore. It transpired that he and his wife had been on a high-protein diet for several months and the pain coincided with that period. He ate no carbohydrates and lived on meat, cheese, chicken, fish and eggs. This could have affected the kidneys and thus the spasm in the corresponding area of the spine (kidneys are embedded in the lumbar muscles). The spasm there weakened the lower part of the spinal muscles and strained the ligaments. I put him on a two-day fruits and water only diet, massaged his spine and gave him some yoga exercises (cobra, semi-bridge, child's pose, arching back, spinal twist). Within 36 hours his condition improved and he was able to walk and sit comfortably.

Jane was a 45-year-old wife of a well-known London businessman. She returned from a trip abroad with excruciating backache. I was contacted immediately. She was bedridden and in agony – sitting, lying in bed, standing etc.

I examined her and it was a case of dehydration and sore kidneys (probably due to excessive wine – which dehydrated the kidneys). She had been in a hot country and drank hardly any water. I advised her to drink a lot of water (two litres a day for 3–4 days) and gave her some simple exercises. Next morning there was no back pain.

Eric, a 65-year-old Danish gentleman, flew over to London to see me. He had an excruciating lower backache, which bothered him day and night. There wasn't a position in which he felt comfortable. There were a couple of disc degenerations in the lumbar region and the surgeons in Copenhagen thought it would be necessary to operate on his back as the pain had been persistent for over a year.

Eric stayed in a hotel over the weekend and I went to see him. The pain was on his left and he could not lie on that side. I tried to prod the area to find out where the pain was coming from but he jumped up as soon as I touched the lumbar region of the spine on the left. Obviously the skin was hypersensitive. I touched various regions around the area and found that the hypersensitivity of the skin was localised in a band across his waist on the left side starting from the centre of the spine. Eric confirmed that his pain was 'burning' in nature. It was obvious to me at that moment that it was post-herpetic neuralgia or severe pain due to complications of shingles. Eric could not confirm any rash on the skin – characteristic of shingles – as the pain started such a long time ago. His MRI scan showed some bulge and degeneration of the three lower lumbar discs but they could not have caused the pain in a higher segment of the lumbar spine.

I prescribed some Zovirax tablets and did some acupuncture. Almost miraculously the pain subsided the following day. I gave him some general treatments in his back with massage and yoga as he did have a mild scoliosis. As he had not done any exercise for a while he had put on some weight so I put him on a weight-loss programme (no alcohol, citric fruits, sweets or desserts, yeast products, cheese, butter, fried food or curries) and asked him to eat slowly.

Eric went back to his country very happy to be cured and much relieved that he did not have to undergo back surgery.

Conclusion

We have just seen that backache usually originates from tendons, muscles, ligaments, joints, discs or bones, but by far the majority of cases are muscular. These are the 'real' backaches originating in the spine. It is also necessary to keep a watchful eye on conditions in other organs that cause backache because these can be misleading and result in misdiagnosis.

Chapter 11

General Treatment

Hippocrates, the father of medicine, by whose preaching I have been greatly influenced, made many major contributions to medicine. The greatest, in my opinion, is the description of the *physis* (I pronounce it 'feesis') or the natural healing power within us. Thus some 2,500 years ago Hippocrates believed and proved that by helping the physis we can help to cure disease and that disease itself is nothing but a sign of weakness of the physis. Some writers later called physis, the 'god within us'. From physis came the words *physician* (one who treats or encourages the physis), *physiology* (study of the laws of Nature) etc.

Hippocrates worked out a simple formula to help the physis. He called it the 'Regimen Therapy'. Common sense tells us that, if we do what Nature expects us to do, we will be healthy provided there are no accidents. Thus, if we eat healthily, sleep enough, do regular exercises, live in a clean environment and maintain personal hygiene, the chances are we will remain healthy and have a strong physis.

Hippocratic Regimen Therapy took account of these essential factors for maintenance of health in treating the diseased state. These factors helped the physis to build up its lost strength to fight a disease.

The importance of this was impressed on me in Moscow where, having completed my medical studies (for an MD), I continued on to advanced medical studies in acupuncture and other complementary medical procedures. Under the guidance of my supervisor, Dr Inna Petrovna Chkalova, I learned to integrate various methods, diagnosis and treatments to get a more accurate perception of the patients and plan a treatment consisting of various modalities of therapy, whose synergistic effect would produce the optimum results. Later, my close association with Professor Yuri Nikolaev, an eminent naturopath in the Soviet Union specialising in fasting therapy and other similar natural methods of treatment, taught me about the latent power within the body to heal itself.

Armed with this knowledge I returned to my home country, India, and began specialising and training in traditional medicines like Ayurveda, Unani, Marma, etc. The scientific analytical format that I acquired in Moscow helped me to understand the methods used in traditional medicine and more so about the way the human body functioned. I was even more convinced that the same laws that govern Nature, rule the body. If we understand it, we can analyse the body's functions and help it to help itself in crisis and disease.

I have used these principles to formulate my principles of Integrated Medical Therapy. It has been divided into two parts: **Regimen Therapy** and **Specific Medical Therapy**.

I have retained the name 'Regimen Therapy' or lifestyle programme used by Hippocrates because it is so appropriate for what it does – puts down a pre-condition, a rule of conduct to maintain a healthy lifestyle.

The **Regimen Therapy** or **lifestyle programme**, which I described in its preventive form in Chapter 8, consists of a dietary plan, exercise and massage:

Dietary plan

This takes into consideration the individual's requirements, food intolerance, nutritional demands, addictions, and the actual disease (hypertension, gout, diabetes, obesity etc). In essence it is moderation and variety that helps the body optimally.

Exercise plan

This is derived from yoga, as it encompasses a complete system of physical and mental exercises. Yoga also covers the stress-management aspect of the

Regimen Therapy of Hippocrates and a separate form of psychological therapy does not have to be included. This is not only an effective way of doing it but is also very cost-effective.

Massage or physical therapy

Hippocrates gave importance to massage, steam baths and hydrotherapy in pools. Healing temples had provisions for these treatments. The Romans, with their famous baths, gave this therapy utmost importance in their lifestyle. It was a place for relaxation and recreation with massages, music, steam and light meals.

In my version of Regimen Therapy, I have included my particular technique for aligning the neck with the therapeutic massage of the entire body. This inclusion makes a world of difference to the healing process as it facilitates the actual healing itself. The sanogenetic process (sanos – health, genos – growth) is geared up to its maximum capacity to aid the body to prevent and fight diseases.

Once the Regimen Therapy is in place, the body and mind have optimum preparation for fighting the disease. It is at this stage that the **Specific Medical Therapy** is applied. These therapies, integrated, produce the best synergistic effect, have an easy run and they work better. If the foundation for healing is laid down by Regimen Therapy, specific medical therapies will work extremely well.

Amongst the specific therapies used at our Integrated Medical Centre in London are:

Acupuncture

Ayurveda

Bio-Energetic Healing (hands-on)

Colonic Hydrotherapy

Conventional (Allopathic) medicine

Hellerwork

Homoeopathy

Nutritional Medicine (including infusions of vitamins and minerals)

Osteopathy, Chiropractic and Cranial Osteopathy

Phytobiotics (use of herbal tinctures)

Psychological Medicine

Therapeutic Yoga

Traditional Chinese Medicine

Unani Medicine

These specific therapies are used to treat various problems either on their own or in various combinations.

For example, if someone has a chronic backache, after the Regimen Therapy is put in place (for weight loss, muscle strengthening, stress management), specific treatments like osteopathy, and acupuncture are used. As yoga forms part of the Regimen Therapy, it can be adapted to cater to the individual's needs in the specific backache – which is why it is referred to as Therapeutic Yoga. This integrated approach not only cures the backache but prevents its recurrence as dietary and exercise regimes ensure that the back is managed well in future.

Regimen Therapy, as described in Chapter 8, is an excellent preventive method as it has all the components of a healthy lifestyle and that is why, at the Integrated Medical Centre, we call the Regimen Therapy a 'Lifestyle Programme'. Keeping control over diet, exercise, stress and circulation, means one is able to maintain health.

Margaret, a 28-year-old woman, came to see me with severe general backache, particularly in the lower back. She had tried different types of treatment and exercises but she had little relief from them. Ultimately she had to take heavy painkillers to give her relief. The surgeons did not find any particular reason to carry out immediate surgery as the discs were more or less intact.

I examined her thoroughly and found the pain localised entirely along the spinal muscles. The tendons of the back muscles located at the base of the spine on either side were particularly sore (thus the emphasis on the lower back). On questioning it became clear that she had several relationship problems and a stressful secretarial job. Moreover, her protein intake was very low (thus depriving herself of vitamin D – the crucial catalyst of calcium absorption

– as well as protein which is essential for muscle-building). I gave her a high-protein diet, coral calcium and relaxation yoga exercises, particularly Shavasana (Dead man's pose). I also recommended general therapeutic body massage, to reduce stress.

Within a few weeks, her backache was better and she was generally very happy.

Stress and backache are closely related. Sometimes people do not need any physical therapy at all to treat their backache. When you go on a holiday and your back suddenly feels better, you know for sure the stress of work has been the main reason for your backache. Good sleep and relaxation can eliminate such backache (stress causes muscle tension and may cause some facet joints to shift or discs to mildly bulge due to the 'concertina affect').

I have derived a range of treatments for backache, based on my observation of the various structures and symptoms. Once again an integrated approach has proved to be the best solution. First, however, I will deal with the general problem of pain.

Pain

There is an important difference between acute pain and dull pain. With dull pain you feel you can make your way through it by lying down, stretching or massaging without doing harm. With acute pain however there is always the feeling that what you do may cause an injury. Acute pain is when a muscle has gone into a spasm, to guard certain areas in the spine where there is potential to do further damage to the back. It is Nature's own reserve system. This is a very sharp pain. It is caused by muscles tightening up severely.

Now these muscles generally tighten because they receive central information from the brain saying you have a tremendous problem there. In this case a group of muscles will tighten up so as to restrict any further movement, because even a millimetre of movement in the spine can cause a nerve to be slightly damaged. Maybe the disc is about to bulge or rupture, so as a warning the muscles go into a spasm. This sort of spasm comes in two main areas:

a

in the groin just above the pubic bone on the side that hurts most, the spine twists because the muscles go into a spasm, and that part you have to massage;

b

in the lateral muscles, which can also go into a spasm. Those are the muscles at the top end side of the seat, and you have to massage the muscles in the spine, which will be very tight.

When you have a pain like that, it is better to lie down on your back and rest and not go against Nature, because Nature is trying to restrict you. Drink lots of water and initially rest flat on the back. Do very gentle yoga so as to slowly and gradually release the tension from the back. If you are able, do some lateral movements sideways, pulling one leg and then the other, because if you are lying down on your back and there is no vertical pressure then the chances are you can readjust the various disalignments. Very often people feel a little click. So it is possible to realign vertebrae without help, just by carrying out these specific exercises.

Help at hand

If there is no help around, that is all the sufferer can do. Let us suppose, however, you are called in to help someone in this sort of pain. You should first of all massage the groin area, then the abdominal muscles, because they tighten up even though they play no role in the maintenance of the back. They tighten up basically to guard. So massage the abdominal area. Use the ball of the palm, and press in the groin area. One side will be more painful than the other; the side that's involved will be very painful, so you massage that area and as you massage the pain will go and if you apply more and more pressure you will tend to get the spine into some sort of order. Then gently massage and tilt sideways in one direction, and then massage and tilt very slowly in the opposite direction.

When possible get the person to slowly turn over onto the front. You must massage the back from the neck right down the entire long muscles. There are short, long and medium-sized muscles in the back, because it has to be able to do various movements. To nod or to bend a little forward uses small muscles. (Note that anterior or spinal muscles with short, medium and long spindles help to bend forward. 'Back muscles' return the body to the verticle position.) To lean forward uses medium muscles. To bend down and pick something up uses long muscles. The short muscles will not permit touching toes. There are different muscles because they have to perform different functions. Bending right down uses a combination of all three.

So you have to massage the entire spine. Right from the top to bottom, toning up and getting rid of all the lactic acid. A spasm in the shoulder area can affect the low back. This is because the neck muscles hold the head. They bear the weight of the head. The shoulder and neck muscles bear the weight of the entire neck as well as the head. The mid-back muscles bear the weight of the shoulders, the arms, the neck and the head. The low-back muscles hold the weight of the entire torso. So you have to make sure that the neck muscles are strong enough to hold the head, the upper back muscles are strong enough to hold the shoulders, neck and head and so on. This is why the lumbar vertebrae of humans are broad and tough, compared to the cervical ones. The skeletal spine is 'conical' to support the weight of the body. You have to make sure that the anti-gravitational forces build up. It's crucial, it is the special part of my back treatment. So you come back to the lateral muscles and the groin muscles, especially when they go into a spasm.

Then you come to the seat muscles and the hamstrings. The seat muscles, the hamstrings, calf muscles and the Achilles tendon, all these posterior group of muscles, play an essential role in preventing the body from falling flat. They are pulling. When you sit on the chair it is only the spinal muscles that keep your erect, but when you stand erect or kneel then the hamstrings, the seat muscles and the spinal muscles keep your erect. When you stand on your feet then the calf muscles and Achilles tendon are involved as well. So you have to massage the calf muscles as well. If somebody is bent over from pain it is impossible to imagine that the seat muscles and the hamstrings and calf muscles are not involved because they are under constant strain. You therefore have to tone them up to bring the spine back into shape.

Posture realignmment

Realignment of posture is the natural way of treating backache. To realign the spine you have to realign the muscles. Fundamentally the back is kept erect by subconscious muscles, which clad the spine. These are too deep to conveniently massage. These strains, aches and pains pass information to the brain saying we are very very tired and tight. Can you do something? The brain then, through the subconscious muscles, adjusts the posture to relieve the pain. So it is the subconscious mind taking control. But it is at a cost. For example if you have backache you do not feel the hamstring muscles. But if you massage them you will find they are very painful. Why? It is the law of dominance coming into force, one pain overwhelming another.

Good posture is when the alignment of muscles and vertebrae in the spine is such that the big muscles have nothing to do because the balance of the spine is perfect. This is often visualised by imagining a kind of puppet string from the top of your head pulling you up, which brings you into balance. This needs to be borne in mind when treating backache. It is not enough simply to massage the larger skeletal muscles, because once the spine is in balance they play no part. The problem is to get at the deep or intrinsic muscles, which maintain the posture. This can be done by very deep massage and you can in fact massage the intrinsic muscles. Massage to the outer muscles results in indirect massage of the intrinsic muscles because the pressure is transmitted through. In fact the result is gentle massage to the intrinsic muscles, which is exactly what they need. The intrinsic muscles, however, are protected, naturally, by the big skeletal muscles so their scope for massage is limited. Another way of toning up the intrinsic muscles is by appropriate exercise, walking on uneven ground, swimming or yoga. Swimming in particular is good for the back because conscious action has to be taken to keep afloat, which brings the subconscious muscles into action. Indeed, well-trained swimming with coordinated breathing is akin to yoga.

Easing tension

When you get backache you panic, which causes tension. Exercising by skilful methods has the reverse effect; swimming in particular produces relaxation of the back muscles. Pain causes panic – be it backache, diarrhoea, stomach ache, headache, these are all Nature's way of warning you. What happens with backache is that, although you have no reason to think you are going to die, you get a tremendous signal to the emotional centre of the brain that something has gone terribly wrong so you have got to take precautions such as lying flat on the back or sitting down. A good exercise in this case is to lie on the back, pull the knees closely towards the chest and feel the back letting go and apparently sinking into the mattress. Do this every half-hour and it is a good therapy for backache. Repeat, relax, repeat, relax. You can actually therapeutically heal your back, if you have pain, even when lying down, because the chances are that it is the seat muscles which are causing trouble, by pressing on the nerve. So if you ask somebody to massage and stretch the seat muscles, then relax, you often get relief.

There is a general tendency to think, 'if it hurts, stop'. This grandmother's rule does not apply to the back. People, especially in the Western culture, have been brought up with the idea that if it doesn't hurt then do it. If it's painful or causing discomfort don't do it. To overcome discomfort, however, you have to allow yourself a little bit of pain because there are no easy solutions (no pain, no gain). So sometimes, when you do exercises, certain areas will hurt because the muscles are inflamed – if you even just twitch it might hurt, there is bound to be some pain. But if you do these movements, in the way the body expects them, you can overcome the pain and there is no harm, provided you are lying down and not doing something vigorous which might rupture something. Gentle movements, even if they hurt, are perfectly all right.

When to seek help

It is safe to try these methods for at least 24 hours before you seek any advice from outside. A qualified integrated physician or qualified therapist will then sort it out for you. But there is a great deal you can do for yourself. Most people heal their backache on their own. In general, if you can find a source of massage, the pain will go away. Some pain is necessary. If you have a known disc bulge then the chances are you are aware of the problem. In that case don't do movements which may be risky. Seek qualified advice. But if the pain is a recent event and not chronic, do not panic. Nature will encourage you to panic but don't. The chances are you can cure it.

If you feel panic the best procedure is to lie down and adopt the Shavasana or Dead man's pose described in Chapter 8. Briefly close your eyes and go through a meditative position. Imagine that your neck is stretching, is being pulled away from your body. You can feel all the tightness disappearing, both in the front and the back. Think of the muscles in the nape of the neck and feel the tension going away. Then feel the shoulders relaxing. Then the upper back. Feel them relaxing and expanding. Imagine them being filled up with blood. And you can see the pain going away. Now you are free of pain in the base of the skull. Then focus on all the tendons and muscles which are very sore, feel them relaxing. Allow them to stretch and relax. Make them contract and feel them shrinking and then extending. Then expand and relax the shoulders. Feel the upper back contracting and expanding. Do that all the way down. Imagine the whole spine shrinking and expanding. As the muscles expand the pain increases, then let go and the pain goes away. You can really feel the spine elongating. This way the subconscious mind will bring about small movements of those intrinsic muscles. Similarly go down to the seat muscles, expanding and contracting. This meditative pose in 90 per cent of cases will relieve the pain. Don't panic but do something. Do it several times a day, using your mind. It is a higher form of yogic meditative exercise. You can with the help of the deeper layers of your mind bring about the twitching of the finer muscles.

Manipulative Therapy

Manipulation by osteopathy, chiropractic and other techniques, when done at an appropriate time, is extremely beneficial. Sometimes the results are instantaneous as the treatment removes the immediate cause of the pain (such as disalignment of vertebrae causing impingement on the nerves).

An experienced therapist will take only a few sessions to resolve the problem and will rely on the body's own ability to maintain the status quo in the back. He will know, however, that frequent manipulation ultimately makes the back lazy.

Always look for an experienced osteopath or chiropractor. The combination of exercises, massage and gentle and infrequent manipulation of the back should take care of the backache. Therapists who insist on manipulation only, and do not recommend any exercises to back up the therapy, are probably not interested in a long-term cure and just want to keep the symptoms under control. Some patients like this kind of approach as it is an easy way out of pain, but it may not achieve long-term healing.

I am often asked what is the difference between an osteopath and a chiropractor. In my view there is a large overlap and each profession has within it a wide variety of practitioners. The differences are largely technicalities. It has been said that chiropractors focus on nerves and bones, while osteopaths focus on soft tissue, bones and blood (circulation). It probably doesn't make a lot of difference because they can't do their job if they don't consider all these aspects. The therapies originated in different countries, they vary in their use of palpation and X-ray in diagnosis, some regard the skull as part of the spine, others don't, but they tend to agree on all the principles I have been discussing. My advice is go to the one with the best qualifications, experience and reputation and at the end of the day probably the one you like best.

Acupuncture

This is another excellent therapy for acute and chronic backache. Sometimes the backache is so acute that massages, manipulation and exercises become impossible to carry out. The patient is in such agony that acupuncture is the only solution. In the hands of an experienced acupuncturist, the therapeutic effect is as powerful as a block with anti-inflammatory drugs injected directly into the muscle. There is, however, no residual chemical to load the liver.

In chronic backache, especially in the elderly, acupuncture becomes an essential therapy in conjunction with massage and exercises, especially when spinal manipulation is contraindicated.

Acupuncture not only removes muscular spasm and pain, but acts as an anti-inflammatory procedure. It should not be taken as an easy way out for 'lazy' people. Exercises must be done to consolidate the effect of relief of pain and discomfort.

Ayurvedic Oil Massage

Hot medicated oils are massaged into the back and rubbed into the muscles. This is done for about 10 days in a row. The anti-inflammatory properties of the oil are particularly beneficial for backache that originates from muscles. Polymyalgia rheumatica (rheumatic muscle ache) is an inflammatory disease of the muscles, mostly affecting the spine. This is a very painful condition. Arthritic type of backache can be treated by this method.

Back Surgery

Back surgery is sometimes necessary, but it should only be considered when other avenues have been tried and failed. If possible, surgery should be postponed for as long as it can be in the majority of cases, but in some the damage to the disc or the nerves they impinge may be so great that it becomes necessary. The following situations are indicative of surgery:

Foot drop

A foot drop occurs when the compression of the nerve roots in the lumbar spine causes nerve damage. It cannot be lifted up as it is paralysed. Surgery can remove the compression, in the hope that the foot will regain its power. In most cases it doesn't, but the sooner the surgery is done, the better chance there is of recovery.

Numbness in the sciatica region

that is persistent and is there all the time. This is also caused by nerve damage.

Rupture of the disc after a trauma

when the compression or fracture is irreversible. The pain and loss of muscle tone should be main considerations.

Severe pain leading to disability

When a patient's life is restricted to bed rest due to severe pain and he is unable to carry out any function, then surgery should be considered.

Loss of power in the hands

and severe pain in the arm and numbness in the fingers which continues. When conservative treatment fails in these situations then surgery is recommended.

Incontinence

A lack of control of bowel movement and urination.

Debilitating pain

which does not respond to any other treatment over 3 months.

Before you go for surgery, prepare your spinal muscles with massages and exercises, for it will take weeks before you can do anything with your back, during which time the muscles might atrophy. Indeed, strict regimen therapy is recommended for as long as possible before any major operation.

Prognosis

Backache can be debilitating. Depending on the individual's threshold to pain, different people react differently. Some people are so impatient that after suffering for a few months they go for surgery. Some neurosurgeons and orthopaedic surgeons are 'knife-hungry'. They do not believe in any conservative treatment, although the acceptance of osteopathy and chiropractic by conventional medicine in recent times has changed the views of many surgeons. Many of them suffer from backaches themselves and are fully aware of the complications of surgery. Even they seek conservative therapy first before deciding on surgery.

Back surgery does not go without complications. As the technology has advanced now, and with keyhole surgery, minimal damage is done to the spine. A new technology is being developed to 'cement' the disc area with a chemical. This means the surgery can be done with the help of a needle and the patient does not need to be opened. Such surgeries will revolutionise complicated backache.

Prevention of backache by maintaining optimum weight, with a healthy lifestyle using Regimen Therapy, is the best solution. Sleep is also a contributory factor. The only time muscles relax fully is when you go into a deep sleep. If you have a disturbed or interrupted sleep the muscles get fatigued. This leads to chronic back-ache. Never underestimate the importance of sleep.

Chapter 12

Conditions of the Neck

Symptoms originating in the Cervical Region

To recap on the anatomical details of Chapter 5, the cervical spine consists of seven vertebrae. The first (top one), named 'atlas', has two major roles to play and its structure is designed to match up to or facilitate the following functions. Firstly, it supports or holds the heavy skull like a bowl of soup and so it has two joint surfaces that are connected to corresponding parts of the skull in the occiput region (lower back of the head). Secondly, it helps to rotate the head. Therefore it has an annular ring instead of the usual main body in the front part of the vertebra, through which passes the projection of the second cervical vertebra and around which it rotates to facilitate lateral movement of the head (see Figure below).

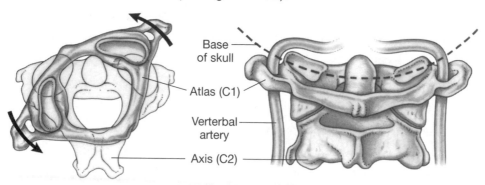

Base of skull

Atlas (C1)

Verterbal artery

Axis (C2)

The second cervical vertebra is called 'axis' because it forms an axis around which the first vertebra and the head rotate. This axis is created by the thumb-like projection of the front part of the vertebra (replacing the standard body of other vertebrae in the spine).

The first two vertebrae are unique because these structures facilitate lateral movement of the head. Although the skull is very tightly bound to the first cervical vertebra by the tough ligaments and powerful tendons of the neck muscles, it can still provide the head with the 'nodding' movement at their pair of joints. As the two vertebrae are extremely mobile relation to each other, they are prone to dislocate causing pain in the lower part of the skull. The powerful ligaments of the occiput often get injured due to falls, accidents, bad posture and whiplash injury. This causes inflammation and subsequent agonising pain in the base of the skull. This pain is aggravated by movement of the head and neck but is generally persistent. Like all tendonitis or inflamed tendons, they hurt most when they are relaxed at night. Thus people with this type of injury frequently wake up in the middle of the night with pain in the occiput or upper part of the neck.

The third cervical vertebra is of particular importance as it is sandwiched between a very mobile second vertebra and a column of relatively less mobile vertebrae (4th to 7th). Whenever there is a sudden movement of the hypermobile second vertebra (axis), the third cervical vertebra is almost bound to be dragged out of alignment. As chiropractors and osteopaths will confirm, this vertebra is the most frequent site for dislocation in the neck. In fact, a few years ago, there was formed a group of American chiropractors which specialised in the manipulation of the third cervical vertebra. They strongly believed that this vertebra was the cause of most neck-related problems.

There are numerous nerves that emerge out of the cervical part of the vertebral column. These nerves innervate (stimulate) the shoulder, neck, arm, hands and fingers. Cervical vertebrae being flat and relatively fragile, often slip out of alignment. Trauma, whiplash injury, falls, using several thick pillows to sleep, bad posture etc can shift these vertebrae very easily. Sometimes the shifting of these vertebrae can cause their discs to prolapse or protrude. These disalignments of vertebrae or disc protrusions can impinge a nerve or irritate it, causing a range of neurological symptoms from pain to numbness in the arm or fingers.

The human neck, unlike that of other mammals, has the flattest and probably the smallest of vertebrae. They are very fragile and thin. As you go down the vertebrae they become bigger. The discs in the neck, however, are very thin, because they only have to bear the weight of the head. Lower down the back they have to bear the weight of the portion of the torso above them as well, so they have to be bigger. In the neck they are more like thin washers so you don't get the same sort of disc problems in the neck. They are layers of cartilage and the internal fluid is minute. (The major disc problems occur in the lumbar area.)

Stress

Stress and overwork cause stiffness in the neck muscles. The tight neck muscles reduce the distance between the skull and shoulder, causing compression of discs and even disalignments of the vertebrae. Certain jobs like using computers all day long, driving for long hours every day, sitting at the desk for hours at a time etc can cause neck stiffness. In this case the lack of movement in the neck not only stiffens the neck but also tightens up the neck muscles. This causes the compression of discs of the cervical vertebrae.

The neurological symptoms that arise out of the neck depend on the type of nerve fibres that are impinged or irritated, and the level at which this happens. If the nerves are not involved then one gets a local pain in the neck and one feels stiffness of the neck. If nerves are impinged then one can feel pain, tingling, burning, pins and needles, numbness and electrical current going along the nerve pathway. These irradiated or referred sensations can go right up to the fingers.

In the embryonic stage, as the arms and hands develop they drag along with them the nerves from the spinal cord there is a link between the two. Therefore nerves are like electrical wires supplying different parts of the limbs and the body. Imagine a man leaning forward and resting his hands on the table. The thumb would be innervated by a higher nerve segment, originating at the level of the third cervical vertebra (C4), because it is closer to the brain. The little finger would get its nerves from the level of the fifth and sixth cervical vertebrae (C5–C6) as it is further down or away from the brain. Thus each segment of the spinal cord produces a nerve that would innervate a section of the limbs. The body is divided into segments and each segment has its own nerve path. That is why, by locating the place where the numbness or tingling is, one can identify the area or the nerve that is being irritated. The simple rule is: thumb is from a higher segment, little finger is from a lower segment.

Pain, tingling and burning sensations arise from irritation of nerve roots by a disc or any other bony structure. Numbness and pins and needles arise out of mechanical impingement of nerve roots that causes loss of sensation. If the motor nerves are compressed, that movement in certain parts of the arm or hands becomes restricted. This results in loss of power in the hand or some fingers.

Common Conditions of the Neck

Arthritic conditions of the neck are quite common and can cause discomfort or pain. If left untreated they can lead to more serious conditions, which are more difficult to treat. Non-arthritic conditions can stem from injury or bad posture and particular examples are restriction of the vertebral arteries, computer ache and whiplash.

Arthritis

There are 14 joints in the cervical spine. These are sites for arthritic changes. The most frequent change that is observed in these joints is a deposit of calcium crystals around the joints. Such calcium deposits can also grow on the edges of the bodies of the vertebrae, just above and below the disc spaces. These deposits are called osteophytes and can be identified on X-rays as spur-like projections. Very often these spurs irritate nerve roots and cause the above-mentioned neurological symptoms.

No one really knows why these spurs or calcium deposits are formed. I personally believe it is connected with our diet. Acid foods like citric fruits, vinegar, white wine, chilli-hot spices etc, when consumed in excess, change the alkalinity of blood or shift its equilibrium to more alkaline. This creates an ideal medium for calcium to be deposited on joint surfaces where wear and tear is great. Just as uric acid crystals deposit in joints to cause gout, calcium deposits in joints can cause arthritis. It can also be said that it is Nature's way of slowing down the wear and tear in joints by immobilising them with calcium deposits, which no doubt produce certain stiffness or restrictions of movements. Wear and tear causes inflammation of joint surfaces. These then become the sites on which calcium is deposited. This usually happens with age when degenerative changes take place or when the neck muscles that hold the head become weak.

Following immobilisation and degeneration the discs dry up and shrink. This causes reduction of blood flow to the disc spaces and degenerative changes take place in them. Similarly joints of the cervical vertebrae can go through inflammatory or degenerative changes. If the cervical joints are inflamed the condition is popularly known as 'cervical spondylitis'. When degenerative changes occur in them, then the condition is called 'cervical spondylosis' (itis – inflammation, osis – degeneration of bones; os – bones). These are very common types of back ache.

The deposits of calcium and other minerals on joint services can grow out of control, appearing like beaks, which can scratch the nerves. This can cause tingling and numbness in the fingers. It can radiate round the shoulders along the nerve endings.

Restriction of the Vertebral Arteries

Aches, pains and tingling are not the only complications of the cervical region. The cervical vertebra is designed in such a way that it has two canals running on either side of its lateral projection (see Figure on page 164). These canals join up to form the vertebral canal, through which passes a pair of arteries and veins known as vertebral arteries and veins (see Figure on page 164). These arteries are the most important in the entire body and therefore they received this special protection of a bony canal. No other arteries or blood vessels in the entire body have had such special treatment in the hands of Nature.

The vertebral arteries supply blood to the base of the brain where all the subconscious nerve centres are. Nature has divided the circulatory system of the brain into two parts. The conscious part of the brain, involved in intellectual, decision-making and logical functions, gets its blood supply through the carotid arteries (the main arteries in the front of the neck). The subconscious part of the brain, involved in the running of the day-to-day affairs of the body, gets most of its blood supply through

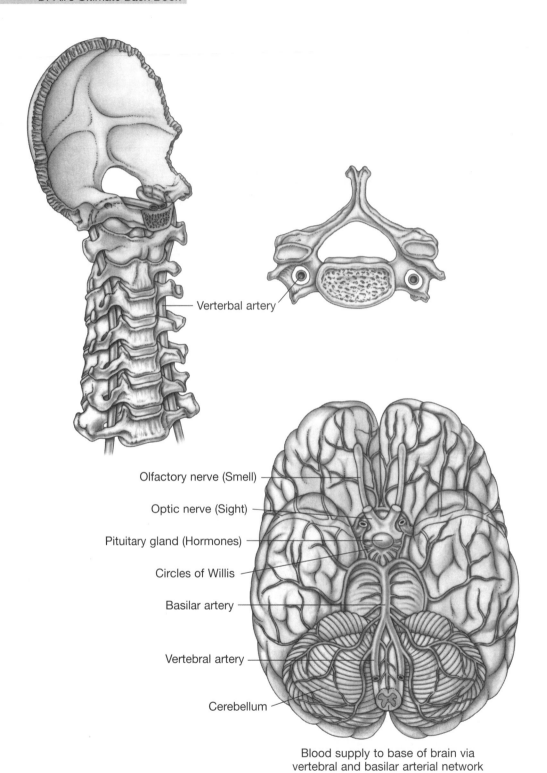

Verterbal artery

Olfactory nerve (Smell)

Optic nerve (Sight)

Pituitary gland (Hormones)

Circles of Willis

Basilar artery

Vertebral artery

Cerebellum

Blood supply to base of brain via
vertebral and basilar arterial network

the vertebral arteries and only a fraction of the supply comes from a branch of the carotid arteries, which does no more than top up the vertebro-basilar blood supply.

The subconscious part of the brain, starting in the brain stem and going up to the area just below the cortex (conscious part of the brain), houses many important nerve, emotional and hormonal centres. These nerve centres include those that control heartbeat, breathing, body temperature, appetite, balance, coordination, muscle tone etc. Moreover, in the subconscious part of the brain there are centres that control sleep, drives (sexual, feeding, thirst etc), moods (well-being or emotion), mimicry muscles (facial expression), swallowing etc. Finally, the subconscious brain also houses the pituitary gland or the master gland that controls most hormones, reproduction, thyroid function, immune system, stress etc. We can clearly see that the subconscious part of the brain controls everything that is necessary to sustain life from heartbeat and breathing to hormonal functions and moods. Therefore, healing this part of the brain can cure most diseases, as this is the well-being centre.

One can do without the conscious part of the brain, as lobotomy (removal of the front part of the conscious brain controlling intellectual functions) and stroke (resulting in the loss of brain tissue in the cortex, controlling movement) have proved, but loss of vital functions in the subconscious brain is life-threatening. The very essence of life is managed by this part of the brain. That is why Nature has provided a well-protected system of blood circulation to this part of the brain. It has left nothing to chance. A brainstem stroke or any damage to this circulatory system (via vertebral arteries) will result in loss of vital functions of life or even death.

Disalignments of vertebrae of the cervical spine can lead to compression of the vertebral arteries. Muscle tension due to stress and strain may also cause disturbance in the blood flow through these arteries. The result is a diminished rate of blood flow to the subconscious brain which will cause the various nerve, emotional and hormonal centres to malfunction. Brain or nerve cells are very susceptible to diminished flow of blood as they do not have any reserve of glucose or energy. They need a constant supply of oxygen and glucose to survive or function; in fact brain cells can survive without oxygen for barely four minutes under normal conditions, after which they begin to die. Decrease in supply of oxygen and glucose may not cause death but will cause deterioration in the functions of the various nerve cells.

There will be a power failure in these cells as a result of diminished blood flow to them, resulting in their poor functioning.

Thus, along with the neurological symptoms caused by neck conditions (stiff neck, cervical spondylitis, cervical spondylosis etc) there may follow a series of other neurological, emotional and hormonal symptoms related to the brain tissue. These symptoms include chronic fatigue, palpitations, hyperventilation, panic attacks, headaches, dizziness, loss of balance, blurred vision, memory loss, lack of concentration, muzzy head, loss of smell, body aches, Bell's palsy, trigeminal neuralgia, blackouts, depression, poor immune system, hair loss, loss of sexual functions, poor hormonal function, loss of libido, menstrual disturbances, impotence, infertility, tinnitus, craving for food or sugar and sleep disturbances. These symptoms appear in a complex about 80 per cent of the time. This collection of symptoms arising out of vertebral arterial circulatory deficiency has been well documented by me and in our clinic it has become known as the ALI SYNDROME (a collection of symptoms manifesting themselves in a group), because I have studied the symptoms over many years and linked them up with problems related to the cervical spine and the vertebral arteries.

I have numerous case histories that logically prove the link between these symptoms and the arteries. By rectifying the defect in the spine I have been able to cure or treat these symptoms, thus proving retrospectively that the two were linked.

Jane, a 35-year-old lady, was diagnosed as having multiple sclerosis (MS) and yet the scans and spinal fluid tap did not show any abnormalities. She had all the symptoms of MS. After a long search for an answer she was sent by me to the Middlesex Hospital in London where a PET scan was done. (These scans are expensive and are offered to NHS patients only in exceptional cases.) This scan showed marked hypoperfusion (decreased blood flow) of blood in the brain stem area. Her symptoms (dizziness, nausea, tingling sensation, loss of muscle power, fatigue etc) matched the findings. Under my treatment she recovered in a few months.

Another example is a typical whiplash injury. Besides the neck injury ranging from pain, stiffness and tingling in the arm to numbness in the fingers, there can also be a range of bizarre symptoms like headache, panic attacks, dizziness, nausea, chronic fatigue, period disturbances, memory loss etc. These latter symptoms, although very subjective, usually do not show up in cervical spondylitis or spondylosis. A whiplash injury shifts the vertebrae and can cause circulatory disorder in the subconscious brain.

Computer-related Neck Ache

As I have said, the neck is a very fragile part of the spine. Moreover, it has to move up, down, sideways, laterally and back. Computer screens, however, are such that you have to keep your eyes focused to meet the tiny flickering letters and if your head moves you can miss something. It has to be stabilized so there is absolutely no movement of the neck, even when you breathe. The letters appear very fast, putting a tremendous load on the hinge joints of the spine. If you overdo it or stiffen the joints, which are designed to move all that time, they get rusty and that's exactly what happens with computer work. Moreover, the head has to be kept steady because it houses the eyes, so the neck muscles have to be so finely tuned that they go into spasm. There is little scope for any movement lest it disturb the focusing of the eye. So the neck muscles are tremendously tight, along with the shoulder muscles and the upper-back muscles. Even the lower-back muscles get very tensed and the movement of the torso can be affected. The neck tension, however, is the most important part. So besides keeping the posture erect, which is done by the finer muscles, the body has been forced by the master, the brain, to keep the eyes focused on the screen. As a result of that the neck goes into a state of spasm.

If the neck is held in that state for several hours a day the chance of exchange of gases and the movement of lactic acid, especially if you're working in a closed atmosphere where there is not enough oxygen, and the oxygenation of these products become very poor. As a result of this a lot of lactic acid accumulates and there is strain of the eye muscles (there are six such groups of muscles) because they are focused at a fixed distance.

In this situation, where the eye muscles are tensed and the neck muscles are tensed and if there is a deadline you have to meet, the stress and the responsibility cause additional tightening of the neck muscles. It is one of the most unhealthy activities that human beings could subject themselves to – much worse than bungee jumping.

You might think that driving is just as bad, but there you look at the mirrors, you look at different distances, you move your head. Driving is highly automatic. When you press your brakes, when you accelerate, you don't have to think. Driving is a most skilful automated activity. On an Indian road where you are constantly over-taking you are under stress, but on a motorway, where most people follow rules, it is less stressful. Knitting is very automatic, very monotonous and repetitive, but you can talk and look up and around. Your neck is not so fixed. Crocheting or embroi-dering is perhaps more akin to computer work. Reading too, even reading in bed for a long time, causes the neck to get tight. Even though your muscles are completely relaxed, lying down, the neck can get tense. With all these you are under control, but with computers you are not and you have the additional stress of avoiding mistakes. Even when chatting on line you are constantly waiting for the letters to come in. But in the banks or in trading you can't make mistakes. You've got to get the figures right. One mistake and they know exactly who's made it. The responsibility can be a killer. As I commented earlier, computers are a noose around the neck of humankind.

A 23-year-old Asian girl in London worked for a High Street bank. She worked long hours at the computer and got very tired. Suddenly she noticed she had double vision and slight loss of vision on one side. Her mother took her to the GP who immediately referred her to Moorfield's Eye Hospital, a leading eye hospital in London of world status. After careful examination and a few tests, a provisional diagnosis of MS was made. The family was devastated as she was to get married within a few months and such a diagnosis in an arranged marriage meant disaster and the wedding would be called off. Everybody was worried. In particular, the steroids that were prescribed did not help at all but on the contrary she felt worse as she had dizziness and occasional loss of balance.

This girl was brought to me for an opinion. Without any comment on her condi-tion, I suggested a course of my treatment. As she had low blood pressure, I gave her a high-protein diet and some B-complex. She received a series of treatments with the Ali Technique and was taught yogic eye exercises to be done twice a day. Her condition steadily improved and a few weeks before the wedding her double vision was corrected fully, and she had no neurological symptoms.

Prolonged ill-treatment of the neck in the above manner can lead to degeneration of the discs and much later on to degeneration of the joints. Both can be prevented.

Whiplash Injury

This is a situation where the control systems in the body, and particularly the posture control system, is taken by surprise. Due to the accident, which is a shock, there is a temporary blackout of all control systems. Your body is first thrown forward and then thrown back (or vice versa in a rear accident). This movement is so quick that the reflexes are not sharp enough and there is inevitable damage to the tendons, ligaments that cover the joints, muscles and the joints themselves. As a result of that you are left with injuries.

When you walk there is a risk of potential injury to some part of the body. Every time you jump from a height there is a potential risk of crushing an ankle or knees and the shock could be transmitted along the spinal joints. The reflex action of the brain, however, causes the shock absorbers in the body to gear up and those which take the load prevent the crushing of joints by creating a gap between the joint surfaces so they don't actually impact. It is the muscles that guard against the shock.

With a whiplash and in accidents that system is overwhelmed. As a result the most common injuries are to the muscles, tendons and ligaments.

There are two reasons for this: (a) at the moment of the impact the tension in the muscles goes beyond the limits of their capability, so they are torn because it is just too large an impact, (b) the complementary muscles are not participating so the main muscles get injured. Thus the main problems of the neck in whiplash are laceration of the ligaments or tendons, which are attached to the muscles, the muscles are themselves torn or strained, and the deeper muscles around the neck also tear because they are too fragile. They carry out finer movements, not gross movements. So the finer muscles get injured most. These are very deep. The actual rupturing of the disc is rare. Sometimes the vertebrae can be dislocated, but usually it is the third joint which suffers torsion. The top two joints are involved in rotation which is not so relevant to a whiplash injury.

Dislocation of the joints, however, carries a complication. The smaller joints are so fragile that this quick dislocation ruptures all the very fragile ligaments that cover them. So in whiplash, even though you might have treatment by manipulation, the joints keep popping out because the actual ligaments had been ruptured, the tissue that holds the joints together. This is a particular feature of whiplash, though you can also get it with chronic postural problems. A further complication is that bad whiplash injury often leads to emotional problems and many symptoms described under Ali Syndrome (see page 173) because of its effect on cerebral circulation together with various other symptoms mentioned above.

Summary

The neck is highly mobile and hence the most fragile part of the spine. It is in itself complex and can impact the brain producing a very wide range of symptoms hitherto never correlated into a syndrome. To do justice to the subject would require discursive analysis of the role of the subconscious brain and indeed justifies a whole book in itself. This chapter must therefore be considered as no more than a preview of the subject, enabling physicians and patients alike to become aware of the ramifications of the circulatory system in the neck and conditions arising from its physical impairment.

Chapter **13**

Treatment of Some of the Common Conditions of the Neck

In treating neck problems the first thing is to ensure is that the nutritional status is right, that is the person should avoid citric fruits, coffee, excessive alcohol, recreational drugs, excessive sugar and drink plenty of water. This is very important. Excessive acid and dehydration, lack of water, can increase the deposits in the neck. Use only thin pillows to sleep, because the more the neck is raised, the more strain there is on the neck muscles when you are sleeping.

Massage

The key treatment of the neck is massage. Start with the shoulder area of the neck, the top of the shoulder. Work over the so-called trapezius muscles, the large rhomboid muscles that extend from the base of the skull, across to the top of the two shoulders on either side, then back along the shoulder blades, converging somewhere in the mid-back area, forming a rhombus. Massage the whole muscle, focusing on tightness in the various areas. Usually there are tight knots on one top side of the shoulder, so you massage this neck and shoulder area, releasing the lumps of lactic acid. Use Dr Ali's Back Massage Oil, and then release tension along the sides of the neck.

All along the sides of the neck, approaching it from the back not the front, you will find very sore body structure. These are the affected joints and they can be extremely tender. Rub them in both directions with the help of the thumb in a rotatory fashion on each of the seven joints. This will not only relieve the pain, but also heal. After this the person should lie on their back. Take a towel and let the neck gently rest on your entwined hands on the towel. Then gently give it a little traction, placing the thumbs just below the occiput, or scalp. Hold it, let the person breathe in and out, and let the head rest on your entwined cupped hands, pulling the head towards yourself, away from the body. Do that for a little while. Feel the neck muscles and massage those that are tight and tender (patients can do much of this themselves). You can easily find the tight and tender muscles, and the more tender they are the more you massage. Gently at first then a little more fiercely later, till you release the tension. One of the signs of the release of this pain is an instant rush of blood into the head and the patient feels good. Then you know the tension in the neck has been released. When muscles are tense they shorten. When they relax they lengthen, easing the pain. You can yourself also use hot tub baths with rock salt, and as you lie in the bath just gently massage the neck area with a little soap. The heat will relieve the tension and the muscles will dilate due to the dilation of the blood vessels. Thus you can easily get more oxygen into these muscles, and the inflammation will go very quickly.

After that you can do a series of yoga exercises, as described in Chapter 8. If you have acute pain you should do the exercises twice a day, morning and evening. In the morning, because that will instantly release the stiffness and will see you through the day, and in the evening, to help you sleep. If it is a chronic pain do it once a day, and have the massages maybe twice a week. Get your partner to do it, or use the self-massage technique.

When massaging the neck area remember the jaws. Pain often causes tightening of the jaw muscles. Release the jaw muscles. The tighter the jaw muscles the tighter the neck muscles. There is a direct correlation between these two. Massage that area, massage the joints, the TMJ joints (the jaw joints), and also massage the temple area just above the ear lobes, the bite muscles. When one is stressed and tense the bite muscles get very tense. By releasing them you release a lot of tension. 'Lockjaw' is a sign of extreme stress.

Specific Treatment

Computer ache: If you tend to use a computer for more than six hours at a time you should try, if not habitually then at least every other day, to massage the neck area and I would suggest that you yourself massage the jaws, the temples and the neck muscles. You have to do it on a regular basis, there is no way of avoiding this. Otherwise it just accumulates. People get panic attacks, tremendous neck tension, they get severely stressed, all because of the tightening of the neck. Even the vertebral arteries become restricted and can cause the Ali Syndrome. If you work at the computer you should take preventive action all the time. Computer neck ache is not usually nerve impingement or the more usual spondylitis type of ache, it is a muscular ache through tightening of the neck muscles. Very often if you swim or do a little exercise it gets dispersed and the pain goes away. But you have to treat it or prevent it, because sometimes working on focal areas cannot release the tension and can result in insomnia-related neck ache. This is a similar type of thing. You toss around, and each time you think of anything stressful, the neck muscles go into a continuous repetitive tightness. Then the flow of oxygen and blood in the muscles is reduced. So you get neck tension, which is basically of the lactic acid type. Always remember that small slow movements of the head do not necessarily distract the eyes, however fixed their focus. The eye muscles work in perfect harmony to retain that focus. Therefore, when working at a computer, small relaxed movements of the head keep both the neck muscles and the eye muscles moving. This is not a complete prevention of the problem, nor does it replace the treatment I have prescribed, but it helps.

Whiplash Injury: Massages and yoga exercises are very important, because they are gentle and they are designed to tone up the muscles involved. They also calcify these areas or help their calcification, where the ligaments have been torn, through local massage. So if you can locate the areas of soreness behind the neck, approaching it from behind and massaging these areas for a few minutes every day, the chances are that they will become indurated or hardened, which means more calcium. The more you rub or provide friction the harder it gets. This helps the ligaments heal. In addition the muscles need toning up, with exercises and massaging. The ligaments, which are deeper, you must also actually massage. You can locate them because the muscles in the neck are in bundles. They are like trees in the forest. So you can bypass them and actually massage the deeper areas, by going between them.

It is stated above that the muscles can be torn. Given time these will heal. Initially it is best just to rest them, with no massage. So with whiplash there are two types of injury. First there is bruising. After the event you are in a state of shock, but 24 to 72 hours later you get an ache. These problems of bruising, torn ligaments etc take a little time to develop. As the phagocytes etc become activated you get various local inflammations. Then you get a further delayed reaction. It could be two months later. This is caused by all the secondary problems, the deeper injuries, discs popping out etc. If the joint is disaligned for a long time, and it is not corrected, then there is abnormal compression of the discs.

The Ali Syndrome: Treatment of the Ali Syndrome requires great skill, normally only accessible through an integrated medical practitioner. Of all the regular therapists probably the cranial osteopath, and the deep tissue massage therapist working on the neck, come nearest.

Indeed, the cranial osteopath in our clinic can claim some success with this condition, not least of all with **Betty**. You remember Betty from Chapter 1? We left her having been diagnosed as suffering a slipped disc, then a dislocated knee, then loose tendons in the knee, then the autoimmune disease, lupus, leaving her a registered disabled person permanently on steroids. It was nearly 20 years later that she came to me a month after surgery. She had suffered continuous bleeding, which could not be stopped and this had finally been terminated with a hysterectomy. Immediately her digestive system ceased to function and she was paralysed from the waist down. I was able to put her digestive system back into action in two days with Ayurvedic herbs and with manipulation and other healing treatment she was walking after two weeks. In six weeks she went horse riding and afterwards complained of being a bit stiff!

Unfortunately her disability had led her to spend hours chatting on the Internet and about a year later she started having dizzy spells and kept falling, on one occasion breaking her wrist. Later she started getting blurred and double vision and occasionally complete blindness. She had to stop driving and for six months, during a savage winter, she was confined to her small flat with constant lethargy, a permanent headache (with continuous prescribed painkillers) and survived largely through the efforts of a friendly neighbour, who looked after her and pushed her wheelchair. Normally a happy woman, despite all her problems, she became depressed and was put on antidepressants. She was taken into hospital for examination, and after a brain MRI and consultations with a neurologist and two rheumatologists (one of whom discarded out of hand a suggestion the vertebral arteries might be involved) they declared they could find no cause for her condition.

She came to me again and this time I went deeper into her background. Her mother had reason to be under severe stress during pregnancy. As a baby Betty had no hair till she was two, a sure sign in my view of a traumatic birth leading to pituitary dysfunction. Later her periods were sporadic, often non-existent and around the age of 30 her ovaries were pronounced to be withered, both conditions, in my view, stemming from the pituitary. A faulty immune system (lupus) also pointed to pituitary dysfunction. Her loss of coordination and balance pointed to dysfunction of the thalamus, failure of the digestive system usually stems from problems of the higher parasympathetic centres, blurred or loss of vision is a problem of the optic centre, depression and lethargy point to the limbic system, and dizziness to the coordination centre in the cerebellum. Where does the nutrition come from for all these nerve centres? You guessed it. From the vertebral arteries.

I adjusted her diet, persuaded her to drink much more water laced with coral calcium, and so reduced her weight considerably and strengthened her bones. I applied my technique to her neck, which at first was agony to her, but after several sessions of gentle massage became manageable and my cranial osteopath took over. Her eyes became normal in a few weeks, the depression and the lethargy went next, she almost discarded her wheelchair and at the time of going to press was thinking of starting driving again and flying off for a holiday abroad.

Chapter **14**

Conditions of the Thoracic Spine and their Treatment

As mentioned before, the thoracic spine is the most stable part of the entire vertebral column. It protects the vital organs within the ribcage and therefore its movement is restricted. It bends a little but twists laterally only marginally so that the ribcage is kept intact. This relative fixation of the thoracic spine does not free it from back pain altogether even though, compared to the lumbar or even the cervical spine, the incidence of disc problems is much lower.

Facet joint dislocations of the thoracic spine are perhaps the commonest form of mid backache. As the vertebrae get disaligned so do the joints between the vertebrae and between the vertebrae and the ribs. The nerves here go in two directions. One part goes to the spinal area and if it is scratched the spinal area goes into a spasm. If it goes along the intercostals or the part along the ribs, then you get pain in the chest.

Most frequently it is the nerve roots supplying the back muscles that are involved and in this case one side of the mid-back muscles goes into a spasm. This pain can be so severe that the person finds it difficult to move or even breathe. The actual impingement or entrapment of nerve roots may happen suddenly (during bending, lifting etc) and the resulting pain is often excruciating and constant. No position can give relief and, unless fixed, the pain is continuous and very irritating. If such a spasm occurs in the upper back then the pain may restrict the movement of the neck and shoulder blade because the trapezius, which is the largest muscle of the back, gets involved and all structures to which it is attached are also affected. Thus movement of the head, neck, shoulder, shoulder blade and upper part of the thoracic spine becomes restricted on one side. This makes the sufferers very uncomfortable as they cannot move or breathe easily.

The other nerve roots that may get involved are the intercostal nerves. The most common site for such impingement to occur is between the fourth and sixth thoracic vertebrae, where the thoracic curve of the spine peaks (see Figure below). As this happens, the pain shoots along the nerve to the chest area and a sharp needle-like sensation is felt in the heart area. This sharp pain is momentary and is connected with the act of breathing which moves the ribs. Very often this pain gets misdiagnosed as heart attack or angina and people are investigated thoroughly only to get negative results.

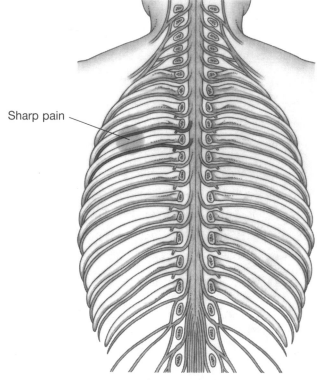

Sharp pain

Intercostal nerves

Disalignments of thoracic vertebrae are caused by trauma, muscle fatigue, bad posture or heavy physical work. Bending over a job or lifting heavy objects is the most frequent cause. Violent coughs and sneezing may occasionally trigger off the dislocation of joints. In these cases the pain is severe and acute. Muscle fatigue due to strenuous and prolonged work may cause pain to develop over a period of time.

Dislocation of the ribs is frequently caused by a fall or sports injury. Although the ribs are securely fixed to the vertebrae, sometimes wrong and sudden movements can budge them out of alignment. This produces sharp or dull pain, which is usually aggravated by breathing. Sometimes people have one-sided posture, perhaps because they are used to sitting in a particular way, so one side of the spinal muscles gets overworked and the other one is lazy. Then the area goes into a spasm. Such people usually have a tendency to slouch over.

Other Conditions

Ankylosing spondylitis

is a back condition which appears in one in 10,000 people. This is an autoimmune disease, which means the body develops 'allergies' towards its own tissue and deposits antibodies (protein particles) on the tissue it 'regards as enemy'. In this case the joint surfaces of the spine, hips and limbs progressively fuse. The disease starts in the neck and spreads downward. The spine joins up like a bamboo losing all its flexibility. It is not until the disease spreads to the thoracic spine that patients and physicians notice the stiffness in the back and its lack of flexibility. This condition causes continuous backache, which is worse in the mornings. The lack of flexibility causes great discomfort, especially when lying down. The thoracic curvature of the spine increases and, in advanced cases of the disease, people become 'humpbacked'. They can never straighten their back, nor can they move their head sideways – everything is fused. This condition may affect other joints such as the hips.

Rheumatoid arthritis

also an autoimmune disease, frequently attacks smaller joints of the cervical and thoracic spine. In this case there is inflammation of the cartilage of the joints leading to swelling and extreme pain. The spine becomes stiff. The pain and stiffness of the spine causes great discomfort to the patients.

Polymyalgia Rheumatica

is a painful condition of the muscles affecting predominantly the muscles of the spine. The spinal muscles become very stiff and painful. Although this condition is called 'rheumatic' it is by no means rheumatism, which is a more debilitating disease. In this case however the pain in the muscles is the overriding symptom.

Thoracic backache

In my practice I have come across several cases of thoracic backache, where the pain starts in the middle of the night. This condition affects people more who sleep on their back. About two to three hours into the sleep the spine begins to stretch and the back flattens a bit. The stretching of the spine allows the vertebrae to move apart. Since, in the thoracic part of the spine, the curvature is greatest, these vertebrae move several millimetres apart as the spinal column stretches. In some cases the movement of vertebrae may trap nerve roots and cause excruciating backache. Once the pain starts there seems to be no relief until the morning when, by standing erect, the curvature of the spine is reinstated and the vertebrae return to their normal positions. Until that happens the pain is continuous and no position can give relief. It returns at the same time every night and patients get very distressed as they toss about in bed searching for a position that will give them some relief. Painkillers are of no use as it is a case of a 'trapped' nerve which is a severely painful condition. A change of mattress can be helpful.

Treatment

The preventive treatment recommended in Chapter 8 is efficacious as a therapy in most cases of mid backache. In the specific case of **thoracic displacement** described above the first thing to try is to lie on the back and relax, though this may be difficult. If so, lie on your front and ask somebody to rub the neck and the spine gently, relaxing the muscles, and ask them to press in the centre of the spine with the ball of the palm starting from the neck region and going down slowly either along the centre or either side of the centre. In 50 per cent of cases it will pop on its own. There will be a slight click and pain will go instantly. But the clicking will depend on how much you have relaxed the muscles. So you must first release the spasms in the neck muscles, because they are also participating, and then release the spasm in the back. It is simply a matter of dislocation of the joints.

Massage and yoga are the best treatment. You must regularly, two or three times a week, have massage with just the ball of the palm pressing these areas until the lactic acid and pain goes away. It is a tremendous relief.

Incidentally, if you do exercises in the morning it is quite normal to get clicks in the joints. It means your spine has the ability to return itself to normalcy, particularly when the facet joints have become disaligned during the night. There is constant slight disalignment of joints which the body corrects all the time. You cannot imagine a complicated structure like the spine moving all the time and not suffering slight distortions, and these are corrected constantly. So long as none of the structures scratch the nerves there is no problem. You could have a very minor condition such as this at any time and you might not know. I regret to say some osteopaths and chiropractors play upon this. The clicking makes a noise, and you think they have performed a miracle.

There is a widely held view that only 20 per cent of back conditions impinge upon a nerve. This is true if you include all these minor disturbances, which don't really cause a problem. If we focus on the back we will find some sort of pain somewhere all the time. There are little pains in our joints and ankles all the time, but if they are below threshold we don't even notice them and they need cause no concern.

For **polymyalgia rheumatica** and **rheumatoid arthritis**, Ayurvedic oil massage therapy (you can use Dr Ali's Back Massage Oil), diet, Ayurvedic and homoeopathic remedies are useful. Acupuncture also gives very good results in these types of backache.

There is no cure for **ankylosing spondylitis**. Symptomatic treatment with massage and therapeutic yoga keeps the spine supple and could even help to arrest the disease. Herbal remedies and acupuncture help to relieve pain and stiffness.

Chapter 15

Low Back Conditions and Treatment

Much of what I have said already applies to the low back. When things go wrong the fault can usually be traced to poor lifestyle, hence weak intrinsic muscles, and the resultant pain is most often derived from muscles, tendons and ligaments rather than discs. There is, however, more emphasis on weight.

The lumbar spine is designed to bear the weight of the torso as well as move sideways. Therefore its components are at risk of damage from excessive weight-bearing as well as the usual muscles related to movement. When the damage is to the discs in the lumbar region it can be traced back to excess body weight, loss of anti-gravitational force due to weak spinal muscles, wear and tear due to age, arthritic changes, stress and strain. The lateral movements of the lumbar spine, lifting heavy weights and the usual injuries and traumas are common causes of lumbar spine injury.

The last two intervertebral discs between L4 and L5 and between L5 and the first sacral (S1) are most at risk. Maximum weight is borne by these two discs. Moreover, the sacrum is fixed to the hip bones while the lumbar vertebrae are relatively mobile and, during turning, maximum strain is put on the last two lumbar vertebrae.

Low backache is a very common complaint. You find it right across the board in adult cases in urban areas. Some people may not be aware of it because their minds are too preoccupied with other things or they do exercises or take precautions on a regular basis. The reasons why backache is so common in the urban area include staying upright for long hours, excess weight, stress, bad posture, injuries or trauma, nutritional deficiencies and genetic factors, conditions I will now consider in more detail.

Staying Upright For Long Hours

Basically the human spine can take only a few hours of strain at a time. If you look at wild animals (except for horses, elephants and other four-legged big animals) they walk, run and rest on their sides from time to time during the day. Chimpanzees, monkeys and gorillas, animals that are closer to the human beings, clearly demonstrate this urge to rest on their backs or sit from time to time. Any physical work can cause strain in the muscles, tendons and joints and the situation demands that one rests those muscles from time to time. Staying erect, supporting the body weight and maintaining posture and balance (when bending, leaning over etc) puts tremendous strain on the muscles of the back. It is strenuous physical work and doing this for long hours at a time that is a serious load on those muscles, tendons and joints. These structures are put under tremendous pressure. They manage the strain for a while and then one day they give up as the wear and tear crosses the threshold to cause signs of disease – pain, weakness, inflammation etc.

Excess Weight

It is obvious that excess body weight will exert more pressure on the discs of the lumbar spine. The excess body weight has to be matched with substantial muscle power or anti-gravitational force to keep the discs intact. If the spinal muscles are weak they create a weaker anti-gravitational force, the force that keeps the spine erect. This results in the compression of the discs to compensate for the weak muscles. As mentioned before, the weakness of anti-gravitational force or the increased gravitational force (body weight) is the main cause of compression of discs. Thus to maintain the equilibrium of discs, the anti-gravitational force must match the downward force created by the body weight.

In space, where gravitational force is absent, there is no pressure on spinal muscles to match with the anti-gravitational force. All the spinal muscles have to do is to stretch the spine to maintain an erect/horizontal position. The discs in this case are completely decompressed or free of any pressure. They retract back to their normal shape in between vertebrae.

Floating in the Dead Sea, where the concentration of salt is high, gives great relief to the back because the discs are decompressed. Floating in water or in a solution (as in Flotation Chambers) counterbalances the gravitational force. The spine feels relaxed. Although standing in these highly concentrated solutions is difficult, the effect of decompressed discs is easily felt in the horizontal position. This relief of pain and tension in the back is more noticeable than when one is lying on one's back in bed. Floating releases all muscle tension.

Thus swimming is considered to give more relief to the back. When standing in water, part of the body weight is neutralised by the upward thrust of the displaced water (Archimedes' principle) upon immersion into it. Everybody has experienced that lifting anything underwater is much easier as it 'weighs less'. This neutralisation of body weight makes the job of the spinal muscles that bear the weight much easier. The apparent loss of weight needs less anti-gravitational force to maintain the erect position. Swimming is therefore considered an easy form of exercise for people with weak back muscles or with disc problems. Nowadays hydrotherapy is used extensively in medical rehabilitation. When muscles are weak, underwater exercises become very easy. It is not uncommon to see patients after back, knee, shoulder and hip-replacement surgeries doing underwater exercises soon after. These patients find it easier to do these exercises in water as the buoyancy helps movement of the limbs. Swimming is also an acquired skill, controlled by the subconscious mind.

Stress

Stress plays a major role in the genesis of backache. In fact, some authors think that it is the only cause of low backache and they are not very far from the truth. Like many other ailments in the body, backache is also exacerbated by stress. As mentioned earlier, stress causes tightening of muscles. The fact that thoughts cause tightening or twitching of muscles has been demonstrated by Mesmer. In his famous experiment, he 'read' people's thoughts by holding their forearms. Thought processes caused twitching of muscles, which he was able to 'read' and 'analyse'. Thus he was able to predict what people were thinking about by feeling the movement of muscles. He carried out various other similar experiments to link muscle activities with mental processes. The word 'mesmerism' was derived from his experiments.

A stressed animal or child has tight neck muscles. This is a defensive mechanism. Stress causes the secretion of adrenalin, a hormone that simultaneously gears up the body for a 'fight' or 'flight' reaction. A rabbit watching a fox nearby has a typical 'flight' reaction, whereas a dog seeing a fox has a typical 'fight' reaction. In both cases, the adrenalin causes increase in pulse rate (heartbeat), blood pressure, breathing rate, body temperature, metabolic rate, glucose levels in blood and above all muscle tension. Whether the animal takes 'flight' or prepares for a 'fight', the muscles tense up in preparedness for the said action. When the situation is changed and the 'flight' or 'fight' motives are completed or aborted, everything returns to normal. This is a physiological reaction.

In a pathological situation, the stress is continuous or the reaction is almost permanent. The body behaves as if it is in a constant state of preparedness for a 'fight' or 'flight' reaction. Pathological stress is characterised by palpitations, hyper-ventilation, panic attacks (a combination of anxiety, palpitation, hyperventilation etc), high blood pressure, insomnia, irritability and of course muscle tension. This tension or spasm in muscles spreads all over from the jaws to the spinal muscles. The body and mind get conditioned like the Pavlovian dogs.

Tension in spinal muscles causes them to shrink in volume and decrease in length to some degree. The continuous spasm of back or spinal muscles, squashes or compresses the discs as the length of the spine is shortened. The tightness of back muscles can increase the pressure on the vertebral column and of course its disalignment at joints or compression of the discs. This is the cause of acute low backache.

As we have seen in Chapter 12, spasm of neck muscles due to stress causes decrease in blood flow through the vertebral arteries. That causes reduction of blood flow to the subconscious brain, the exact anatomical area that houses the centres for muscle tone and involuntary centres that control erect posture. Thus the muscles that stretch the spine upwards lose their power and the vertebral column loses its power to remain erect. As a result of that, scoliosis sets in. In fact most scoliosis in children is caused by the stress factor. They have abnormal spasms of muscles, which distort the normal curvature of the spine.

This loss of power in the upward-stretching muscles that maintain the erect posture, reduces the anti-gravitational force, which could be another reason why discs compress with stress. This, however, happens in the chronic stage when the stress factor is permanent and its effect is overwhelming. This is the cause of chronic low backache. Thus we can see that stress can cause acute and chronic backache, depending on the period through which they exist. Acute stress causes instant tightening of muscles and compression of discs. Chronic stress causes impaired functions of posture-maintaining nerve centres, which ultimately reduce the anti-gravitational force resulting in the disc compression.

Posture

Posture plays a very important role in backache. All the major organs of the body are located in front of the spine, in the chest and 'belly'. There is nothing at the back other than spinal muscles and the skin. It is because of this odd distribution of weight that the spinal muscles at the back have constantly to pull the body over like a pulley unless held in a state of perfect balance by good posture. There is, however, a constant tendency for the body to stoop over or fall forward because of the weight of the organs. This forward-bending force is counteracted by the pull of the spinal muscles. This happens automatically because of the 'stretch reflex' (referred to earlier). Therefore in the erect position, the back muscles and all the muscles of the back portion of the legs (gluteal or seat muscles, hamstrings, calves etc) are in a state of continuous strain unless good posture is maintained. That is why 90 per cent of muscular sprains in the body occur in the posterior part.

If one leans over or lifts weights all the time, the back muscles and the associated muscles of the legs are under increased pressure. They simply have to work that much harder to keep the body erect by pulling it back. Once in the vertical or erect position the other force, namely the anti-gravitational force, takes over and maintains the posture. Thus anyone who leans forward or sideways, either at work or otherwise, is jeopardising the back muscles and making them vulnerable to injuries and strains. The more the strain, the more the inflammation there is in the muscles and tendons.

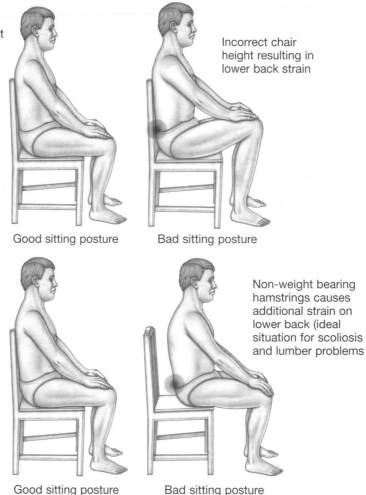

The body's weight supported by gluteal and thigh muscles relieving the lower back from additional strain

Incorrect chair height resulting in lower back strain

Good sitting posture   Bad sitting posture

Non-weight bearing hamstrings causes additional strain on lower back (ideal situation for scoliosis and lumber problems

Good sitting posture   Bad sitting posture

This is often apparent to a golfer practising putting for a long time. This action of course weakens the spinal muscles, causing disc problems eventually. The only safe position for the spine is an erect posture. Anything that makes it bend forward or sideways would, after a period of time, lead to spinal problems. Bending forward repeatedly and over long periods of time will injure the back muscles. Leaning sideways will strain and weaken one side of the spinal muscles or the other. If one leans more to the left then the left side of the back will hurt more. Bad posture engages the superficial muscles continuously which then maintain the bad posture and cause the deep intrinsic muscles, which should be maintaining the posture, to atrophy, weakening the anti-gravitational force. It is a vicious circle resulting inevitably in backache.

In the vertical position, the spine carries the body weight and the axis through which it transfers weight runs through the axis of the lumbar vertebrae and the sacrum. If the body tilts to one side then the axis moves away from the centre of the spine, laterally to the same side. In this case the weight is borne by a part of the sacroiliac joint on the same side, instead of the lumbo-sacral joint in the case of a perfectly erect posture. This causes injury to that side of the sacroiliac joint. This joint is forced to bear the weight of the torso when it is not meant to. Thus the sacroiliac joint can get inflamed and cause lumbago and one-sided pain.

The above pain forces the spine to twist or curve abnormally, in order to compensate and to try to reduce the pain. This results in twisting of the lower back and hip area, which is very noticeable.

The Alexander Technique, a method of posture regulation, pays a lot of attention to the way one sits, stands, walks etc. The emphasis is on keeping the spine aligned and erect through various posture-regulating techniques. In fact Alexander himself believed that stress, poor well-being and discomfort in the body are caused by poor posture. Nerves that regulate the body emerge from the spine and therefore he believed that looking after the posture was the single most important thing for a person's well-being.

Yoga assigns a lot of importance to posture. According to some masters, the four most important parameters of health are: good posture; sound sleep; good appetite; and clear bowel movement. Therefore a healthy person would have a good posture, standing erect and with perfect alignment of the spine. This ensures the body feels good. Bad posture is a sign of illness or poor well-being. It is not surprising that people stoop, slouch in chairs, walk badly etc when they are not well or very tired.

Injuries or trauma

A large number of backache cases stem from injuries or trauma.

Sports injury

is the commonest form of trauma the spine receives. Amongst the different varieties of sports that cause low-back injury is squash. It causes low backache in almost all cases as it involves bending too low to pick up the ball and turning quickly. The ball moves at great speed as it rebounds from walls, which are only a few feet away from the player at any given time. The game puts one's reflexes to their maximum test and the two players must be at risk of running into each other as the court is nothing but a small confined space. Fast, vigorous, sudden and abnormal movements put the spine at greater risk than almost any other sport. Other high-risk sports like horse riding, weightlifting, tennis, etc have their own problems. Those who are involved in such sports usually get injured when they are either very fatigued or when their muscles are not toned up enough before the sport. The risk of injuries increases with these conditions. Fatigued muscles or weakly toned muscles easily become traumatised. Periods of rest in between strenuous exercises are necessary, otherwise the risk of repetitive strain injuries increases.

Strenuous jobs

such as lifting, carrying and standing or sitting in one position for a long time at a stretch increase the risk to the lower back. As mentioned before, lifting weights makes the lower back arch forward while the upper back leans back as if to carry the weight on the chest. This increases the curvature of the lumbar spine, putting the lumbar, especially the last lumbo-sacral discs, at risk and under great pressure. Such activities traumatise these discs by weakening the ligaments that bind these vertebrae and ultimately dislocating them at the joints.

Weight-related injuries

These arise when a person puts on a lot of weight. It is well known that most excess fat in the body is accumulated in the belly area. This is because the belly area is fairly inert or does not work that often. When mammals walked on all fours their bellies had to have powerful muscles to 'hold' the abdominal organs in place. Since Homo Erectus, or the first man who walked erect, the abdominal muscles have had to have just enough strength to keep the organs in place. Most of the weight of these organs is borne by the spine and the pelvis in the erect position. Thus in human beings the abdominal muscles have become more lazy or inert. The abdominal surface becomes an easy spot for a deposit of fat, which generally likes sluggish parts of the body and hates being moved about too much. Thus we have fat deposits on the face, under the jaws in the neck area, bellies, sides of thighs, below the arms etc.

Another favourite spot for fat deposit is in the omenta or sheaths of ligament that bind the intestines together and suspend or support them. If these ligaments did not support the intestinal mass it would slump on the pelvic floor on account of its weight. In fact all organs, such as the liver, spleen, uterus etc, are suspended by their own ligaments. These hold the organs in place. When the groups of ligaments of the intestines (omentum) have excessive fat deposits they become very heavy and put additional pressure on the abdominal walls. This is the origin of the 'abdominal bulge', when the belly sticks out. The sheer weight of the internal fat (in the omentum) and the external fat deposit on the outer wall of the abdomen make the belly 'billow' out and move down to create the sail-like bulge. 'Beer belly' is an example of such a tummy. This puts tremendous pressure on the lower back as it is forced to curve forward to adapt to the weight it has to bear. Thus weight gain and the adjacent bulge of the abdomen strain ultimately damage the structures of the lumbar spine.

Nutritional Deficiencies

Bones, muscles, ligaments, tendons and cartilages are part of the body. Even though bones seem to be a 'dead' part of the body, they too need nourishment all the time and suffer if it is diverted. If the absorption of calcium from the colon is poor, either due to a lack of it in the diet or due to Irritable Bowel Syndrome and other gut conditions, the concentration of calcium in the blood drops. Muscles need calcium to contract or else that function will be impaired. Such muscular organs as the heart would not be able to function properly if the supply of calcium was not adequate. Thus a reduced level of calcium in the blood will force the body to steal the element from bones, where it is deposited in abundance. This is the cause of the washing away of calcium from bones, known as osteopenia (os – bones, poros – holes) or brittle bones. Osteopenia – when calcium loss is marginal; osteoporosis – when calcium loss is great.

Muscles, ligaments and tendons are active tissues. Movements in the body would not be possible without their participation. Therefore there is a tremendous wear and tear in these tissues. These need constant repair and that is not possible without nutritional adequacy. Proteins, minerals and glucose supply have to be continuously maintained in these tissues for them to function properly. For example if a weightlifter did not eat enough proteins, his muscles would not be able to regenerate or repair themselves. Sumo wrestlers eat up to three kg of meat or chicken a day to maintain their muscle bulk and tone. Boxers too need a certain amount of protein and carbohydrate supply on a regular basis.

Similarly a supply of potassium, iron, cobalt, magnesium etc is also essential for maintaining the wear and tear in these soft tissues. As mentioned earlier, tendons have microscopic blood vessels that supply them. These are essential for their functioning. Since nutrition is an essential part of all living tissue, lack of it will cause them to malfunction or ultimately necrotise or die. Except for hair, nails and to some degree the outer part of teeth, all tissues need nutrition to survive and function.

A big South African rugby player came to see me at my friend Johann Rupert's holiday home near Cape Town, where I go in January every year. This was a young man, very fit, and yet his lower back and groin pain made him skip important games. The surgeons were contemplating a minor surgery to suck out one of the discs, which showed a bulge.

When I met him I knew instantly that he could not have any disc problem. Firstly the pain in the groin and his low backache could not be linked as the concerned disc (L4–L5) would only send pain, if it did, along the sciatic nerve path, i.e. the buttocks and side of the leg and not in the groin (usually L1–L2 zone).

I began to question him about his diet and lifestyle. He was stressed because he was only 22 years old and was playing in the top team. The main problem was his intake of citric juice (eight or more glasses of very acid orange juice, 'to increase vitamin C'), white wine, nuts etc, which caused excess stomach acid (he had heartburn). Within a few days of avoiding acid foods (citric, spicy, nuts, alcohol) and prescribed painkillers (also producing stomach acid), he was cured.

Traditional Indian medicine always points out that citric fruits are bad for aches and pains. In my experience, I find the acid-producing food (in the stomach) makes tendons, ligaments and joint surfaces hurt more as they become inflamed, the skin surface becomes spotty, the wine causes a burning sensation in the bladder and urethra, and generally makes one tired and unfit. The exact mechanism of this reaction of the body to acid food is not known. It must be due to some chemical reactions that take place in the body – such as the collagen fibres becoming chemically destroyed. Collagen is an important building material for joints, ligaments and tendons etc.

Genetic factors

Sometimes genetic factors leave the spine with some defects that cause an ongoing back problem. **Spina Bifida** is a typical example of this. In some babies the posterior arch of the vertebrae, especially in lumbar area, fail to join at the centre, and a gap results between the two arches (spina – spine; bi – two; fida – branches). In this medical condition one can see a gap in the spine in X-rays. This can often be felt from the back. Depending on the size of this gap and location of this defect, various types of spinal and neurological symptoms occur. Some people live with it all their lives without realising that they have spina bifida. Others have pain in the back, poor development of leg muscles, weak gait etc as the nerves from the spine are affected.

Scoliosis is also considered by scientists to be a genetic problem. Often it runs in families and this gives them the reason to think that this is a genetic disorder. In my opinion scoliosis can also be caused by extreme stress, insecurity in childhood as well as nutritional deficiencies during the growth period. Thus it is a multifactorial health condition.

Diagnosis and Treatment of Low Backache

Just to summarise then, the low back is more prone to injuries than any other part of the back. It bears the weight of the torso, the architecture is completely wrong for a human being standing erect and the low back is forced to carry out certain functions for which it was not intended in the chain of evolution. So there is great potential for problems. Moreover the discs are big, they take a lot of shock when we walk, when we run, when we jog, and the abdominal cavity has a tendency to put on weight, emphasising the unusual distribution of weight. There is a tendency for the stomach to bulge out, putting extra load on the lateral muscles and abdominal muscles to keep them intact. If they are not exercised then they put secondary strain on the back, and the back muscles, especially the lower back muscles, are placed in tremendous tension using the entire system to try to keep the whole spine erect. If, on top of that, there is additional weight, then the tendons of the spinal muscles get very sore. So most of the backaches in the lower back are from these tendons and muscles, and not usually from the discs.

If it is a disc problem then there is likely to be irritation of a nerve, which will cause pain in the direction of the nerve. Just as an electrician knows where the fault is in an electrical circuit, similarly a good physician or intelligent layman will know where the fault is in the spine. Disc problems will always cause irradiating pains in the lumbar region. Certain nerve fibres go straight to the actual spinal muscles and some of them follow another path, as in the case of intercostal and mid back pain. Just as we saw in the neck, certain fibres go straight to the back of the neck, others divert down the arms.

Problems of higher lumbar joints

If the nerves that are scratched, irritated or compressed go along the lower part of the body, then you can get pain in different directions. The higher nerves will go to the groin area, while the lower they emerge the more they go to the side. (Take an animal on all fours. The nerves of the big toe and front of the leg come from higher segments, while those in the small toe and back of the leg come from lower segments.) If you get a pain in the big toe or the groin or inner thigh then the chances are the fault is higher up. The lower down you go the more lateral it is. That is the general rule. If it is the outer toes, the little toes, then it is lower down. So if it is on the outer side it is lower down, inner side it is higher up. If everybody knew this, patients would not panic, but it is something that doctors don't tell you. So if you get pain in the groin and inner thigh then it comes from lumbar 1 (top lumbar) or lumbar 2. If it is much lower or to the side then it could be from L4 or L5. The nerve from L1 and L2, besides going to the groin also goes to the thigh area, so if you get a burning sensation when you touch the thigh area, if your slacks irritate the skin, which is too sensitive, then you know there is a problem with L1 and L2. Now those two areas rarely go out of alignment. Because the higher [you are – 'it is'?] the less the chances of it being displaced. This is because maximum compression takes place between L3/L4 and L5/S1. These are very close to the powerful sacrum bone, and that's where maximum weight is. So if it is higher than L4, then consider this: (1) have you drunk enough water? The kidneys are embedded in the lumbar muscles. If they are dehydrated they weaken the muscles in that area, resulting in all sorts of pain, which can actually press on the nerve or push a vertebra to irritate a nerve root. (2) If this is not the problem, then ask someone to massage you in that area and there could be instant relief from the sensitivity and the pain in the groin.

Lower joints

If the lower discs of the patient are affected, then you have to be very careful. You go down from the tail bone area and just where the actual vertebrae start there is a flat sacral bone (see page 61). You must try and massage just on top of the sacral bone. It will be very very tender, because that is where all the tendons of the muscles are attached. The whole point is the entire transmission system of the muscles acts as one in the places where they are attached and in the main bulk of the muscles. If there is any defect or pain in any of these structures right from the neck down to the sacrum then it is going to affect the spine somewhere. The patient has to be pain-free and injury-free. The spine must be in a straight line laterally. In scoliosis things go wrong because the spine is not in a straight line. So that area must be massaged. Just above that area these tendons of the sacrum converge into two very tight tendons of the long spinal muscles. This is the key. They come in like your arm, and they diverge like fingers over the bones. So this is where maximum pain is. When you talk about lumbago pain, this is the type of pain. It is a typical ligament-tendon-muscle pain, with nothing to do with discs. So rub that area and especially rub and give friction heat and use your palms to apply Dr Ali's Back Massage Oil and rub it. The more heat you generate the better. Tendons have poor blood supply so the more heat you generate the more the blood is encouraged to flow. When you rub it you not only displace all the chemicals and lactic acid but you allow fresh blood to accumulate in the area so the tendons heal. Tendons love to be rubbed and with the friction heat they heal. While cold compresses and ice packs take the pain away temporarily, they numb the pain, but they do not participate in the actual healing as constriction of blood vessels has little effect on inflammation. Heat is what tendons and muscles love, to dilate, to allow more blood to flow. So you massage that area and very often the pain is completely relieved just by massage.

Irradiated pain

Now if you go higher up on these muscles, literally about one to one and a half inches (depending on age and size), from the central axis (the bony bit), and you keep pressing upwards you'll find one or two areas that are very sore. These are the discs. To correct that, place your thumb against the central axis and gently push it in the opposite direction, on each of these three or four vertebrae. This is where, if the discs are involved, it will hurt and it will show you exactly what level the problem is. Then use the massage, because of the guarding effect, to tone the abdominal muscles. Massage the seat muscles, and the muscles of the hamstrings. If it is a sciatica, i.e. pain going down the outer area, then there are two most likely causes: (1) the actual nerve has been irritated by scratching from the discs and the different bony structures, or deposits which can be corrected by yoga; (2) the seat muscles have gone into a tight lump, either due to overuse such as standing, lifting, carrying or through constant sitting. (When you sit down it is the seat muscles that bear your weight.) So you must massage that area deeply. This lump or knot of muscle is actually pressing on the sciatic nerve, which comes out from the abdominal or pelvic cavity into the outer surface of the leg. That's where it emerges. If you massage that area and the lactic acid is dispersed, there is less pressure and an inflamed nerve can then heal very quickly (if there is pressure there is less blood flow). If, however, the nerve is inflamed through diabetes or other conditions, then of course the patient should let it rest and take vitamins and minerals and look after their general health. That's what sciatic pain is all about. Sometimes these 'knots' in the seat muscle are from irritated nerve roots of the L4–S1 area.

Sciatica

To treat sciatica you massage all the seat area and behind the knee, where there is a tight muscle called the poplitea, whose nerve comes very close to the surface of the skin at that point. If the muscles behind the knee are very tight they can also press on the nerves. Relieving this spasm brings relief. Any osteopath who treats such conditions without paying attention to the state of the muscles is making a mistake. You should spend a lot of time softening up the muscles, and making sure there is no damage done. A tightened or inflamed muscle is more susceptible to injuries, so violent manipulations can tear them up. A good osteopath will spend 10–15 minutes of the time massaging and softening up all the muscles that are involved in the actual guarding or pathological reflex since when there is pain, the body guards it. If you massage that, then do a gentle manipulation and you'll find that the manipulation has a long-term effect, very often after only one treatment. But if you don't prepare the body then you often have to go back again and again. Next time you go to your osteopath or chiropractor ask him or her to massage the spinal muscles and give you some exercises. In my opinion those who comply are the more conscientious.

Conclusion

Low back pain is characterised by the failure of the spinal muscles to support the body's weight, either because that is excessive or because the muscles are out of condition. Naturally prevention is recommended, by adopting a healthy lifestyle, in particular by doing the daily exercises in Chapter 8. When things go wrong, however, the fault is generally muscular and much can be done by yourself and your partner. Common sense diagnosis and massage is infinitely preferable to spinal fusion.

Chapter **16**

Secondary Diseases
of the Spine

Self-help for backache is wise before seeking professional treatment. When the need arises, however, the lack of gatekeepers (or true general practitioners) in national health services or conventional clinics means that you are going to have little guidance on which professional to choose. It is therefore important to understand that the cause of backache does not always originate in the back. It can arise from secondary diseases. By secondary disease I mean that the main reasons for or causes of the various spinal problems lie elsewhere in the body and the back is the unfortunate victim of the primary disease. These conditions arise out of the malfunction of the rest of the body and the disease may not have originated in the structures of the spine in the first place. Hence optimum treatment is not necessarily available from a back specialist, though it still might be.

Autoimmune Diseases

Rheumatoid arthritis is a typical example of this type of secondary spinal condition. This disease attacks the different joints and connective tissues of the spine and various other parts of the body. The body develops some sort of 'allergy' towards these tissues and attacks them with antibodies. That is why it is called autoimmune (auto – self) disease.

Polymyalgia Rheumatica

This is a common disease of the muscles, particularly those of the spine. The principal symptom is muscle ache (poly – multiple, myos – muscle, algia – pain) in different groups of muscles. The pain probably gets aggravated with cold and damp conditions, like rheumatism (rheuma – cold and damp). This disease is also an autoimmune type but in this case muscle tissues get 'attacked' by antibodies. The muscle ache in the spine, especially in the early hours of the morning, can be unbearable.

Secondary Cancer

It is not uncommon for secondary cancer to appear in the spine. When a cancer spreads from its primary site (lungs, colon, prostate, uterus etc) it can lodge in the bones of the spine and form secondary sites. These islets of 'secondaries' spread into the bone tissue and cause tremendous pain. Sometimes the pain is so unbearable that morphine is given periodically to dull it. These back pains are continuous, stabbing and are mostly localised. They cause discomfort in movement as well as when lying still.

Pregnancy-related Backache

This is usually caused by the strain on the muscles and ligaments of the lower back. The increased weight in the front part of the spine creates a tendency for the body to bend forward rather like someone with a 'pot belly' (putting on weight with overindulgence in food and alcohol). The pulley system of the spinal muscles in the back is geared up to counteract that force and pull the spine erect.

Many orthopaedic surgeons and even physiotherapists and osteopaths explain this phenomenon differently. They say the tummy 'bulge' moves the lumbar vertebrae forward causing 'lordosis' (curved forward) and thus the impingement of nerves resulting in pain. From my own experience, in cases of 'lordosis' or forward bending of the spine and 'kephosis' (backward bending of the spine, as in 'humpbacks') there is hardly any pain. Somehow these movements seem natural to the spine as in bending forward to lift, carry or do a job and leaning backwards to look up. What the spine does not like is twisting or bending laterally or sideways using the oblique or waist muscles. In these movements the small interconnecting joints of the vertebrae ('facet joints') are more likely to dislocate or go out of alignment.

Moreover, on simple examination of the spine in pregnancy or abdominal-bulge-related lower backache, I have always found the lumbar muscles to be taut, strained and tender. The tendons of the muscles attached to the sacrum or the lowest part of the spine are extremely tender and inflamed. Treating these with massage, heat and exercises eliminates the pain in a vast majority of the cases, thus proving retrospectively that they were the cause of the backache and not the shifting forward of the vertebrae.

Towards the end of pregnancy, in preparation for birth, the pituitary gland in the base of the brain (the 'seat' or control centre of thyroid, reproductive and stress hormones) secretes oxytocin, the hormone that eventually causes contraction of uterine muscles or labour pains. This hormone softens up the joint of the pelvic area by creating 'controlled osteoporosis' or 'brittle bones'. As this happens the pelvic girth is ready to enlarge and allow the foetus to pass through without serious complication.

Sometimes, due to nutritional problems and the strain of the birth, the softened bones and joint surfaces do not heal very well after the labour. In such cases the women are left with some residual pain in the lower back, which can persist for months. Massage and good nutrition can eliminate these pains in most cases.

The larger the baby the more complicated the pregnancy-related backaches become.

Constipation-related Backache

There is a possibility that chronic constipation can cause some referred pain. That is to say, hardened stool masses create obstruction to the passage of gases and the overstretched bowels may cause colicky pain, which can be felt in either the lower abdomen or lower back. Most constipation-related backaches are constant and dull in intensity. Sometimes they remain there even after the bowels have moved, either naturally or aided with enema/colonic hydrotherapy. Such prolonged pains are caused by a completely different factor.

Calcium, magnesium and other minerals are absorbed only in the colon. Iron is absorbed primarily in the stomach (that is why people get anaemic after stomach operations or with ulcers or gastritis). Now chronic constipation, chronic diarrhoea, ulcerative colitis and other inflammatory bowel diseases cause lower calcium absorption. After a period of time the muscles which need calcium to contract will steal it from the bones, causing mild or severe osteoporosis. The pelvic bones, being large and porous, become vulnerable and the calcium loss from the joint surfaces of the lumbo-sacral region causes inflammation and pain. Unless the calcium level is reinstated the problem will not be eliminated overnight. Thus chronic constipation or bowel-related problems cause a nagging low backache for a long time, unless the calcium returns to the bone. The ache or severe pain can continue as in the case of osteoporosis. Steps to improve calcium and vitamin D intake described above should be taken.

Old Age Low Backache

Ageing causes osteoarthritic changes in the facet joints of the lumbar spine. These inflamed joints (caused by wear and tear) may hurt on their own. The discs of the lower lumbar vertebrae may degenerate and dry up. This causes the vertebrae to sit one on top of the other without the cushioned disc. The absence of discs may not cause any pain as such or else everyone who has had a disc-removal surgery would complain of severe pain. What one feels is stiffness and perhaps restriction of movement around that area.

One of the commonest forms of backache in the elderly is caused by scoliosis. Due to weakening or wasting of spinal muscles, the anti-gravitational force is reduced to the very minimum, and so the spine shrinks and acquires an S-shape configuration to maintain the vertical posture. Such deformations lead to irritation of nerve roots, muscular spasms etc, which generate pain.

Another common cause of backache in the elderly is the atrophy or wasting of the seat or buttock muscles (known as gluteal muscles). It is the firmness of the muscles which bears the weight of the torso in the sitting position. When these waste away, due to age or fatigue, the buffer zone is reduced to a minimum and one ends up sitting on the sacrum or the hip bone (pelvic). Those joints (sacroiliac) begin to be traumatised and hurt. This sort of pain is very annoying and usually gets worse as more trauma is caused by the weight-bearing activity. Sometimes the seat muscles are so wasted that people sit on their sacrum and coccyx tailbone. This often leads to excruciating pain in the tailbone area, especially while sitting. I have seen patients who had been wrongly diagnosed by specialists linking such pains to degenerative changes in the lower discs and advising surgery. Most people after a certain age have such degenerative changes, but this may not be the cause of pain in the sacrum or tailbone or low back. A simple examination of the 'seat muscles', helped by a bit of logic, would reveal the source of such pain in the lowest end of the spine.

Salman, 57 years old, had suffered from back pain and 'sciatica' continuously for two years. Normally if he stood up, walked or lay down, he would be okay, but his pain would start below the right thigh soon after he sat down. His scans showed a mild bulge of the disk between the L4–L5 (lower lumbar disc). When I examined him, there was not much tenderness in the lower back area or the seat (gluteal) area but his hamstrings in the right leg were tight and slightly tender. I asked him to describe his back pain again.

It transpired that his pain started 10–15 minutes after he sat down on a chair. The pain would gradually increase till it was so unbearable that he had to get up and walk, when it would be relieved in a few minutes. Sometimes, if he was sitting at a formal dinner, he would squeeze the under surface of his right thigh to get relief. The pain, however, would persist. This was so inconvenient that he would walk up and down his office and lie on the sofa to give dictation. Sometimes he would spend the entire working time sitting on the edge of the table in the vertical position or standing. He avoided formal dinners and socialising as much as he could. He had seen all sorts of specialists, osteopaths, acupuncturists, healers, physiotherapists and magnet therapists, but had no real relief. Finally he decided to get surgery on his back as was suggested by his neurosurgeon.

I asked him if he was a keen sportsman before. He said he used to do a lot of exercise and gave it up a few years before. I asked him if his leg muscles had wasted as a result of that and he confirmed they had. Here was the main clue – muscle atrophy. When muscles waste the fibres lose bulk or protein – they do not disappear in their numbers as most people think. You are born with a finite number of muscle fibres, they only become bulky from within with protein. So when muscles are not used for a prolonged period of time many blood vessels collapse and are replaced by fibrous (scar) tissue, making the muscles hard. Now, when Salman sat on a hard surface (e.g. a chair), the wasted hamstrings were squashed due to his body's weight. The already reduced blood vessels could not cope with the demand for oxygen in these muscles. When one sits the weight of the body is borne by the contraction of the hamstrings and seat muscles on both sides. Thus decreased blood flow caused accumulation of lactic acid and subsequently the muscles went into a spasm (like a cramp). This was the origin of the pain. Standing up and walking or squeezing the muscles would give relief or eliminate the cramp and pain.

I massaged the hamstrings very deeply and told him to eat carrots (to give potassium) and take extra calcium (deficiency in either or both can cause cramps in muscles). He was also recommended some yoga exercises designed to strengthen the back and stretch the hamstrings (semi-bridge, half-swing, boat pose, child pose).

With this treatment his pain initially became less intense and the duration for which he could sit before the pain started increased until the pain completely disappeared.

In this case I did not treat Salman's back at all. His problems were not related to the back or the lumbar discs, which had only a mild bulge. Surgery in this area would not have given him any relief. This is an example where all irradiated pain in the leg is blamed on lumbar discs. There are exceptions and doctors should diagnose each case with utmost care. At age 50 or so most people would have some disc bulges or degeneration in the lumbar region, which might not be scratching the nerve to cause pain.

Injury to Buttocks

Sometimes younger people can have pain in the lower back when they fall on their seat and the muscles or the tendons of the seat muscles attached to the sacroiliac joint get squashed. Tendons heal very slowly as they have weak blood supply (that is why they are white in colour), so when they are injured or inflamed they take a long time to heal. Therefore soft-tissue trauma of the hip area (as in a golf swing, gymnastics, landing on the buttocks after a fall or slip etc) can leave a prolonged agonising pain in that area. These are purely soft-tissue (muscles, tendons, ligaments) injury and have no neurological connection (due to disc prolapse). In fact these pains have nothing to do with the spinal column.

Ed Moses, the athlete who won all 400m hurdles for nine consecutive years (including the Olympics) had his entire career ruined by injury to one such muscle segment in the seat area during a miscalculated twist. For several years he was misdiagnosed and treated unsuccessfully for a back problem until I had a look at him during a Dunhill golf tournament. It was such a relief to him to find the true cause of years of suffering.

Tendonitis

The long muscles of the spine (known as the erector spinae) end up in a pair (on either side of the spine) of tendons, as all muscles do, but these are very thick and powerful. These tendons are attached to the outer surface of the sacrum, as most tendons (except the mimicry or facial muscles, which are attached to the under surface of the skin to produce facial expressions) end up on bone surfaces. Strain injury of powerful tendons caused by lifting heavy weights or by doing repetitive jobs or bending sports (squash, tennis etc when you 'pick up' the ball again and again by quickly bending down and rising to the feet very quickly), cause excruciating pain in the very bottom of the spine in the lumbo-sacral region (fifth or last of the lumbar vertebrae and the first sacral vertebra or fused sacrum). This tendon pain is diagnosed as lumbago, which is a purely tendon or ligament pain and has no link with the spine. Sometimes a cold draft or exposure to a sudden chill due to inadequate clothing can cause this inflammation. This causes spasms of the tiny blood vessels on these tendons (heat-preserving reaction of the body) and initiates an inflammation pain (chilblains are another example of pain caused by inflammation due to blood-vessel constriction on exposure to cold).

Lumbago

Many practitioners think that lumbago (or pain in the lower back spreading across the small of the back) is caused by sudden 'prolapse' of the last disc of the spine just above the sacrum. This is not true, as this area, bearing the bulk of the body's weight, has very little scope for movement. Moreover this last disc quickly 'solidifies' into bone in adulthood in a majority of cases. Even if there were a disc prolapse there are no nerve roots in the immediate vicinity as the spinal cords disperse into nerves leading to the foot and leg at the level of the third or fourth lumbar vertebrae (see Figure below). The nerves at the end of the spine near the sacrum are like a bundle of loose electrical wires and no mechanical protrusion or disc can scratch or irritate them. In the upper part of the spine these nerves emerge out of the spine as nerve roots, which are perilously close to the discs of the various vertebrae. Lumbago is a diagnosis which orthopaedic surgeons or doctors rarely make today because it is vague 'unscientific' terminology. Moreover they do not quite understand its origin and explain the cause in terms of discs or nerve roots. Lumbago is a colloquial expression rather like 'crick in the neck', 'brittle bones', 'shingles' or 'hayfever'. They do not really fit into the medical description of things. Therefore lumbago has come to mean simply an acute low backache localised in the lower part of the spine.

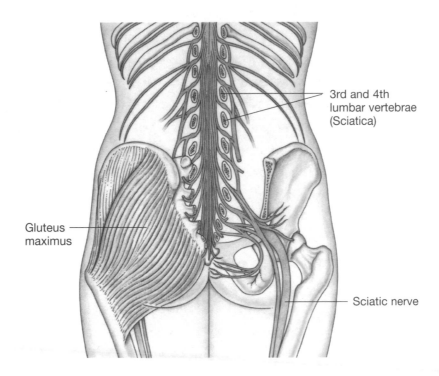

3rd and 4th lumbar vertebrae (Sciatica)

Gluteus maximus

Sciatic nerve

Piriformis Strain

Underneath the layers of muscles of the seat (major and minor gluteal muscles) there is a strong strip of muscles which is attached to the head of the femur bone. This muscle is called the piriformis. It is a delicate muscle and is often prone to injury due to sudden movement of the leg (football kick) or repetitive movements like hiking up mountains or working on a step machine. An injury to this muscle takes a while to heal because it is relatively delicate. Inflammation of this muscle causes a dull but annoying pain in the seating area on one side. As there are many layers of muscles over it, the pain is often misinterpreted as a disc-related radiating pain from the lower lumbar region. Unless somebody physically probes deep into the seating area to actually locate the strip of often hardened muscle (in spasm due to inflammation), it cannot be easily identified. It remains a hidden cause of the pain in the hands of inexperienced physicians or specialists, who are obsessed with scans and X-rays, which do not show signs of inflammation of soft tissues like muscles. This is an example of the importance of hands-on examination of patients in medicine. Ironically it can be treated with massage of the affected area (described in detail in Chapter 13), hot poultices and exercises.

Inflamed Hip Joint

The seat or gluteal muscles are attached to the top or head of the femur (the thigh bone) in the hip joint area. These muscles together with muscles of the thighs help to move the leg around the hip joint. Therefore when the hip joint is inflamed, as in osteoarthritis, traumatic and rheumatoid arthritis, these seat muscles contract permanently to restrict the movement of the hip joint. It is Nature's own way of controlling pain and further damage to the joint surfaces. The gluteal muscles become tender and inflamed in the process. Inexperienced physicians often wrongly diagnose this condition as (additional) back problem, especially if they do not probe the seating area or do not see the logical connection between the two. The body always reacts to an injury or damage with some symptoms or other. This is the rule of Nature. Massage, as described above, is the best treatment.

Cysts

Over the past 20 years, I have seen a handful of cases where low backache had been caused by cysts under the sacral bone or within the body of the sacrum or around the nerves that ultimately form the sciatic nerve. Cysts are benign bubble-like growths with fluid inside. The pain is either due to its direct mechanical pressure on the bone's surface or due to irritation of the membrane of the cysts during bowel movements and gas. The pain is projected on to the lower back. Such pains are throbbing by nature. As the cyst grows the pain increases. Its surgical removal is a complicated procedure and surgeons do not always recommend it. They prefer strong painkillers or even morphine to surgical intervention. Homoeopathic remedies could be used instead of surgery.

Conditions of Pelvic Region

Numerous conditions of the pelvic region, like endometriosis, bowel cancers, bowel diseases like fissures (cracks on the walls of the bowels caused by extreme dryness, constipation etc), haemorrhoids (internal), fistulas (infected tunnels originating in the bowel and penetrating into the surrounding tissue and harbouring pockets of pus causing excruciating pain and discomfort), irritating contraceptive coils in the uterus, etc cause pains which, although originating in the internal organs of the pelvic region, often project themselves on to the low back. Treatment for all these conditions should be obtained through the conventional GP.

Asymmetry

Sometimes people are born with legs of different lengths. This is not unusual as there is always an asymmetry between the right and left side of the body. In an eye test the vision is different in the two eyes in a large majority of cases. Hearing tests often show differences in the two ears. However sceptical scientists may be, the two arms and legs are often different in size and length. It is not uncommon to see the two thighs of different size because of the favoured use of one more than the other. Sometimes a right-leg user may have weaker thigh muscles in the right (probably a genetic or developmental problem, or a nerve degeneration).

The difference in length between the right and left legs causes asymmetry in the hip alignment and subsequently the spine. This causes mild to moderate spinal scoliosis (lateral or S-shaped curvature of the spine). Once that happens the centre of gravity of the body shifts from the middle of the joint at the base of the spine to one or the other sacroiliac joints (between sacrum and the hip bone). The shifting of the weight-bearing axis from the centre (along the spine and straight between the legs) to one side puts unusual strain and pressure on the muscles and joints of the corresponding hip and leg, resulting in inflammation of the joints, muscles, tendons and ligaments. This can lead to pain in these structures. One-sided backache, sciatica, osteoarthritis of the hip and knee joints are not uncommon. Spinal scoliosis stemming from conditions other than differing leg-size, such as bad posture, nutritional deficiency, extreme stress, trauma, degeneration due to osteoporosis etc can also lead to displacement of the weight-bearing axis and cause similar one-sided pain in the low back, sciatica, osteoarthritis etc. The cure is normally special shoes, but the treatment for the pain is massage.

When there is a problem, discs of the lumbar spine usually bulge on one side or the other. This bulge leads to spasm of muscles on the affected side and disaligns the spine and distorts the posture. People with acute or chronic backache are thus tilted to one side. One shoulder is lower than the other and one hip is raised. This is a temporary scoliosis of the spine and as soon as the condition is treated by massage and the pain subsides the spine returns to its more normal alignment.

Sometimes the spasm of muscles could be in the region above the groin or pelvic bone. Such spasms or injuries would be due to sports (picking up balls during tennis and particularly squash games, football kicks, sword-fencing etc) or by carrying heavy weights with one hand. These localised injuries could be sub-threshold, that is to say strong enough for the brain to interpret but not strong enough for the conscious brain to register (just like in a massage one discovers areas of spasms and pain in the body which otherwise lie dormant). To protect and adapt to the latent area of pain and spasm, the hip can twist forward or sideways, causing disalignment of the spine. Very often I would treat these painful areas of the groin or lower abdominal muscles just above the pubic bone, and this would automatically align the spine to eliminate low backache. This I discovered using simple probing of muscles during treatment and using logic to explain the origin of disalignment of the lumbar vertebrae and the corresponding pain.

Postoperative Backache

When surgery is contemplated, the backache being treated usually originates from the discs. When bulging or after rupture they can scratch or compress nerve roots causing severe pain, tingling, numbness and muscular weakness, depending on what nerves they have damaged. Now, logically speaking, when the pain returns after surgery, it is right to assume that either the original pain was not caused by the discs or the new pain does not originate from the discs. In the former situation surgery was not the right solution or treatment, and in the latter the surgery did not cure the backache and probably created new complications. If there is no disc (scooping this out is the most common surgical procedure – either in part or whole) then where is the pain coming from?

The most common cause of post-operative backache originates in the muscles and tendons. In the absence of the natural 'shock absorbers' or 'buffers' (discs), the muscles and tendons take up these functions while walking, jogging, coming down stairs etc. This repetitive strain causes muscles and tendons to ache, due to lactic acid accumulation caused by excessive demand of energy by overworked muscles. This may often lead to inflammation, which causes symptoms like early morning stiffness, chronic pain that does not go away with rest (ache caused by lactic acid disappears with rest), restriction of movement etc.

Sometimes scar issue is formed around the site of the operation and this may extend to the nerve roots and cause permanent pain. This type of complication may lead to continuous pain along the direction of the nerve and get projected on to the areas where these nerves end (toes, calves, groin, sides of the leg etc).

Sometimes surgery involves fusion of vertebrae with metallic plates. This causes almost total loss of mobility of the spine in that area. Discs are scooped out and plates, nuts and bolts are put in the necessary areas. When bones later degenerate, either due to age or nutrition, these metallic parts may become loose and touch sensitive muscles, nerves and ligaments causing moderate to severe pain. I know of a scientist-businessman who is fascinated by the latest in orthopaedic surgery for treatment of back and shoulder problems. He has had more pains and agony from screws and nuts going loose from bone degeneration then from the actual disease.

I met **Robert**, a 40-year-old healthy gentlemen, at a dinner in Cape Town. He was in such agony that he could barely sit on his chair. He had recently had back surgery, where a 'wedge' was put into the lowest disc of the lumbar spine to fix it. Top surgeons performed the operation and it was done with great care. Unfortunately the pain in his lower back persisted. It was obvious to me (as it is in so many cases) that the disc was not the original cause of his backache. I offered to see him the following day.

His old scans confirmed that he had a disc bulge in the lower lumbar spine. On examination I found the entire area around the scar very sore. Surgeons pull the skin and underlying tissues apart to make a gaping hole so as to carry out their job. When stitched back they leave a thin scar covering all the evidence of the underlying tissue damage. The result is often painful scar tissue and poorly healing bruises, which unfortunately hurt.

On manual examination, I found the tendons of his long spinal muscles (erector spinae), over the place of attachment on the sacrum, extremely tender. It seemed to me that his low backache was caused by these inflamed/injured tendons and perhaps not the discs. In the vast majority of cases, disc-related pain spreads across to other regions. Localised pain (as in lumbago) originates from muscles, joints, tendons, ligaments and the actual vertebrae.

I explained what the situation was and asked him to come to London for a couple of weeks for treatment. Here I treated him regularly, massaging the sore spots, and gave him gentle yoga exercises to improve his flexibility. Within two weeks he was perfect and a couple of months later he resumed his golf – a passion for him.

Four years later he had to move house. While doing so he had to carry heavy boxes. As his back was perfect and well-maintained, he had completely forgotten about his back problems. Suddenly the back 'snapped' and he was in great agony. He collapsed. After resting in bed for two weeks he went to have an MRI scan which confirmed a bulge in the disc above the one that was fixed by surgery. He had sciatica and was very poorly. After three or four months he made an appointment to see me in London. I said I would do my best to alleviate the pain, warning that if he was not careful it might come back. He was put under our treatment. After a week of massage and yoga his sciatica disappeared but the back pain persisted. He began to supplement the treatment with a couple of hours of exercises at the gym.

One day at the yoga therapy session one of the stretches caused a snap in his spine and the pain came back with a vengeance. I advised immediate rest at the clinic. It was obvious that the excessive exercises had indeed fatigued his muscles. Yoga is largely very gentle and done with utmost care, but there is a golden rule: you must rest the muscles after yoga for up to 24 hours. Somehow, vigorous gym exercises are not suitable for damaged spinal structures. The pain was excruciating so we had to inject some anaesthetic-anti-inflammatory complex to numb the pain.

A scan was done and it did show the prominent bulge appearing in the previous scans. I advised him to undergo keyhole surgery (minimal damage) to remove the disc. If the treatment had given him relief by retracting the original bulge, the excessive exercises probably undid the benefit and the bulge was back.

As he was well rehabilitated with massage and exercises before the surgery his recovery was miraculous. The keyhole surgery eliminated his pain and the general condition of his back helped him to spring back to life within a couple of days.

Was surgery avoidable in Robert's case? My answer is no. After the first surgery he probably did the same thing that caused his back trouble. His personal problems had caused him a lot of stress and fatigue. Gym and excessive exercises were not the right solution – stress management was. Moreover, the first back surgery destroyed the natural 'immunity' of his back. As is always the case, back surgery creates imbalance in the anti-gravitational force by forming scar tissues, restricting natural movements of the spine and creating a renewed awareness of the affected area, causing postural problems. All these factors created abnormality in Robert's spine and its posture after the surgery.

Backache Due to Standing in Erect Posture

After a heavy day's work, standing at a cocktail party for an hour or so becomes an agony for many. Such people look for empty chairs, of which there are few, to sit down and rest. These pains start after standing in one place for a few minutes. The ache gets worse as time goes by and then becomes unbearable.

Most doctors that I know seem to think this pain is caused by a degenerative disc. I disagree with them in a majority of cases. Such pains disappear when sitting down or moving about or walking. If it were purely disc-related, then it would continue to hurt in a sitting or moving state, because the disc would continue to bulge, if it were weakened, in all vertical positions. Walking or sitting down should not eliminate the pain. In fact walking might aggravate the pain with movement.

The real reason for the pain is muscle fatigue. Weak muscles get tired more easily only because they do not have full weight-bearing capacity. Such muscles have poor blood supply and therefore oxygen is not available to the muscles to meet their demand. Lactic acid is formed and the muscles begin to ache. After a while some muscles give in because very little oxygen (or energy) is available to them, thus reducing their anti-gravitational force. This may lead to secondary compression of the disc and complications like acute sciatica-like pain may follow. A bit of massage (to improve blood flow), a bit of rest by sitting (to let the lactic acid get metabolised by oxygen) and a bit of movement (to improve blood flow to the muscles) eliminates such symptoms very rapidly. Standing is more strenuous than sitting because in a sitting position the seat muscles (gluteal) do not participate in the generation of the anti-gravitational force from below the hip area. Moreover while sitting one uses the backrest and arms if available, which give an additional support to the spine by taking on some of the load. The best treatment is exercise (see Chapter 8) to tone up the posture-maintaining muscles.

Backache While Lying Down

There are three areas of the spine which can hurt when lying down. This depends on the problems at the upper-back, mid-back and low-back areas. These are usually caused by displacement of vertebrae. As soon as one lies down, the spine is stretched as the various curves acquired from forward-bending, bad posture or trauma are modified. As the vertebrae move around the nerves are pulled with them and this results in spasms of muscles and subsequent pain.

Amongst the pains caused by lying down is a specific one, mentioned earlier, manifested in the mid-back area. People with misalignment of vertebrae of the mid back, about two to three hours after falling asleep, wake up with excruciating pain in the mid-back area. The body gets used to a certain posture during the day, but when lying down the natural adjustment of vertebrae produces discomfort and pain. Once that happens, the pain doesn't go for several hours as the sufferers change sleeping posture several times, looking for a comfortable position, till finally they fall asleep. Their sleep is therefore disturbed and patients get very agitated because the spasms and pain return every night like clockwork. This may last for several months. Such cases are best treated with manipulative therapy (osteopathy/chiropractic). Similar pain may be observed in people with mild or moderate back problems when they lie flat on the carpet (see MOT).

When lying down, the seat area on one or the other side may press on the sciatic nerve which emerges out of the lower abdominal cavity in this particular area. The seat or gluteal muscles, especially if they are tight knotted due to strain, injury or inflammation, are pushed up, pressing the thick sciatic nerve and causing severe pain locally (more so when it is inflamed) and sending electric currents down the side of the leg and to the little toes. Sometimes one may feel numbness or cold sensation depending on the type of sensory nerves compressed.

Sometimes, similar pains may arise from the nerve root irritation by discs protruding at the level of the fourth or fifth lumbar vertebrae. Lying down may stretch or move the fragile vertebrae and bring about these symptoms.

Severe mid backache may cause great distress and agony in patients suffering from hiatus hernia. They may wake up in the middle of the night with this pain. Wind in the large intestine or gas in the stomach may push up part of the upper stomach into the weakened part of the diaphragm, near the point of penetration of the oesophagus (food pipe), causing herniation and entrapment. This pinching of the stomach wall causes severe pain and may project into the mid-back area. Unless the herniation reverses, the agonising pain may be persistent. Occasionally intake of anti-acids and loud burping may relieve this pain.

Gallstones, pancreatitis (inflammation of the pancreas), pleurisy (inflammation of the membrane of the lung), stomach ulcers etc frequently project pain on to the mid-back area. These pains are distinguishable from genuine spinal problems by the fact that physical therapy or manipulation does not relieve this pain in any way. Only the elimination of the main cause of the projected pain can bring about relief.

Very often dislocated rib joints cause severe pain in the mid back. Contrary to general belief, ribs can move. This is noticeable during breathing. This movement of a rib is possible because of the joint where it is attached to the vertebra. Trauma is the most frequent cause of dislocation of this joint and once that happens very precise manipulation is required to put it back in place.

Backache Related to Vegan Diet

One sees many people who have become vegetarians nowadays. Strict beliefs about not eating flesh out of regard for living things should be respected as an individual's and not as a universal choice. These people often do not know how to balance their intake of protein. With widespread intolerance to milk products, the matter has become more complicated. Lentils, nuts, cheese, tofu (soya) etc have become the protein source for vegans or vegetarians. These proteins do not contain the fat-soluble vitamins, such as vitamins A, D, E and K. These fat-soluble vitamins are present in animal fat and lack of vitamin D in particular leads to malabsorption of calcium. Moreover, protein is an essential transporter or carrier of such elements as iron and all other minerals so it is an essential building block. By depriving the body of protein, the daily wear and tear, such as that which takes place in the back and neck or due to computer injuries for example, does not heal well. A survey done by GPs in England showed that 65 per cent of Indian vegetarians, for example, have osteoporosis by the age of 65. That is indicative of what goes on. Protein is essential, especially for the spine and the bones in temperate countries where there is a lack of sunshine and vitamin D synthesisation is limited. The short gloomy days of winter cause deficiency in vitamin D and hence calcium. In India however, where there is a lot of sunshine, the level of osteoporosis in vegetarian women is not high. Traditional dresses that cover most of the body when going out may be the contributory factor as vitamin D synthesis is lowered. Lack of sunshine combined with constipation is a dangerous combination. Vegetarians should eat soaked almonds (soaked for 24 hours – change water several times) and protein supplements, do regular exercises and have mustard and sesame oil body massage, especially after the age of 50 years.

Conclusion

Backache can result from a variety of causes not related to the back. Hasty recourse to back treatment should therefore be avoided until careful analysis and diagnosis of the symptoms has taken place. Much of this is well within the capability of the individual and guidance has been given above. Even when one is convinced that the back itself is at fault, 24 hours of self- or partner treatment is normally well worthwhile before professional help is sought.

Chapter **17**

Prognosis

Mark, 65 years old, was recommended to me by a well-known interior designer friend of mine. He was about to go for spinal surgery and wanted a second opinion.

Mark had burning pain on the upper surface of the right thigh, especially above the knee. This area was extremely sensitive to touch. Even if his trousers touched this area, the pain was intolerable. The pain was continuous but worsened when he stood up and walked. He was on many painkillers including high doses of Tegretol, a medicine used to suppress epileptic fits (which are caused by abnormal electrical activity of the brain) and severe pain. Mark's scan showed that his last two discs of the lumbar spine (L4–L5 and L5–S1) were degenerated (not unusual for a 65-year-old), and the surgeons wished to target these. I knew the surgeons were wrong and would not have given relief to Mark's pain. If these discs had been the cause of his agony then this pain would have been irradiated or projected along the path of the sciatic nerve, i.e. the side of the thigh and leg, and down to the right little toe, but not on the top surface of the thigh. Pain or numbness in this area originates in the root of the nerves in the upper lumbar vertebral region and typically the discs between L1–L2 and L2–L3 would have caused it. Many orthopaedic surgeons make this blunder as they 'see' bones, not nerves.

The matter seemed to be as simple as following the electric circuit in a house. If there is no electricity in the kitchen, why should the fuse of the bathroom be changed or its circuit replaced?

I touched and prodded Mark's upper lumbar region on the right – it was extremely sore. On questioning he confirmed that he hardly drank any water and was drinking too much wine and some coffee. All these must have affected the kidneys and so the soreness in the upper lumbar region. The tightness of the lumbar muscles in this area felt like a lump ('knot'). This focal tightness must have been irritating the roots of the L1 and L2 nerves by the shifting of these vertebrae. That explained the pain.

I changed Mark's diet to exclude coffee, salt, alcohol, yeast products, red meat, sugar (to make him lose some weight), citric fruits and spicy food. I asked him to drink two litres of water per day. I massaged his entire back, starting from the neck, right down to the low back, toning up the muscles and especially pressing the sore lumbar area on the right with the ball of my palm. Then I gave him some yoga exercises (cobra, child pose or pawan mukt asana, swing, semi-bridge and arching back) to be done twice a day. The same night he had some relief and two days later his pain had gone. The first thing he did was to cancel the surgery, annoying the surgeon at one of the leading hospitals in London. I saw him quite regularly for a month and he was cured. Today, ten years later, Mark continues to have a normal life, doing his exercises and drinking more water.

To my great surprise BUPA happily paid all my bills, something they rarely did if you used anything other than conventional medicine, especially if you are not registered with them as an approved 'specialist' by their panel of doctors. (I had been refused enrolment as their specialist on an earlier application some years before.)

Backache is conventional medicine's major weakness. Medical colleges do not provide adequate physiological knowledge or background to equip doctors to treat it. The nutritional content of their course is inadequate. They are not taught any but the most rudimentary palpatory techniques, which are absolutely essential for the treatment of the back. They are not taught the theory of exercise so they normally do not know how to put their patients on the road to recovery. As far back as 1986 *Which?*, the monthly magazine of the then 600,000-member Consumers' Association, surveyed 4,000 of their members who had tried complementary medicine. 81 per cent had unsuccessfully tried their GP first. 82 per cent claimed to have been cured or improved (31 per cent cured) by complementary medicine and the problems for which it was most commonly sought were pain back pain or joint problems (71 per cent).

How has this come about? It did not happen in Korea where medical colleges put all their physicians through the same syllabus for the first few years then allow them to diverge into traditional or conventional medicine, both of which are treated equally in the national health policy. In Hong Kong and Thailand there have been shifts in this direction in the medical colleges. India has achieved the same result by having conventional, Ayurvedic and Unani colleges providing courses of similar length then recognising the graduates on equal status. Integrated medicine (the culling of the best from all forms of medicine), was developed in Russia and China during the 20th century and is now well established there.

In Western countries more and more conventional doctors are seeing the shortcomings in their education and are either studying complementary subjects or freely referring patients to complementary therapists for treatment they know their own modality cannot economically or safely provide. It has been reported that in Britain the 36,000 GPs are now outnumbered by around 50,000 complementary and alternative medicine practitioners. As the case of Mark shows, there is even a chink in the armour of the insurance companies.

It all came about like this. Conventional medicine began in Europe as an alternative to traditional medicine about 300 years ago when it was realised that its development had been repressed by the Church for a thousand years and was now sadly trailing behind countries such as Persia, India and China. They used, as a shortcut to catch up, new developments in science that appeared to offer ways of predicting reactions of the body instead of learning from the experience of their forefathers. This was fine to start with. They did catch up and in some ways (but not others) overtook their traditional colleagues – but at what a cost. The science they depended on was concurrently developed to produce a huge array of chemical drugs, without their long-term side effects being properly assessed, to produce a huge array of expensive advanced technology that diverted physicians from the diagnostic skills of their forefathers and broke the vital doctor–patient relationship, and to produce an insurance industry with the financial resources to support the enormous cost of those drugs and technology. Because of the colossal finance involved governments were forced to provide budgets and regulations not previously needed when medical ethics were the controlling factor. (The 2,500-year-old Hippocratic oath is still used at graduation today, but stands as little more than a symbol in our modern society.)

So we have conventional medicine now harnessed to four huge financial monoliths, governments, drug companies, technology and insurance. Doctors no longer enjoy the freedom to practise the art of medicine. They are virtually forced to do it the way these monoliths dictate, though not, as I say, in Asia, Africa or Russia which constitute more than half the world's population. Conventional medicine is still the minority modality. Life expectancy is still longest in the world in Japan and Hong Kong, not in the countries tied rigidly to conventional medicine. The result is that inexpensive techniques, such as diet control, massage and exercise, though safest and most cost-effective, are not encouraged because, to put it bluntly, there's no money in them – no 'meat'. But these are the pillars of backache treatment, which is why it has become conventional medicine's greatest weakness and why it has become such an enormous drain on the resources of urban society. In a study a few years ago in Canada an association of hospital administrators discovered from extensive research that if low backache were referred to chiropractors in the first instance instead of GPs, it would be safer for the patients and would save Canada $30 million every year.

Backache stands as the shining example of the weaknesses in conventional medicine. The failure generally, not to focus on the three vital parameters – physical and emotional health, stress management, circulation and digestion – has led to an incipient weakness in the whole of conventional medicine, provoking misdiagnosis, iatrogenic illnesses, and above all excessive cost, so that we now have to face unsustainable health policies, appalling waiting lists for treatment (patients even dying in the corridors of A & E departments in hospitals before they can be seen), critical shortages in medical staff and even the export of patients abroad for treatment. On the other hand patients themselves are seeking better conditions and treatment, are trying to treat themselves with supplements and aerobic exercises without adequate knowledge of how to do so in the optimum way and, thank Heaven, doctors themselves are breaking their shackles and introducing common sense into their practices. Even scientific research is beginning to unearth evidence, particularly in the field of bio-photons and bio-communications, for the life force and healing power within us, previously regarded as mythical by conventional medicine, and there is a glimmer of light that mysteries such as acupuncture and homoeopathy might have a scientific explanation after all.

Medicine has, I believe, started on the long long road to recovery, against the tide of the financial monoliths. What can we do in the meantime?

I believe there is a lot we can do. Chapters 7–9 give some sound advice on how to keep a healthy back for life. If schools were to take up the challenges and make healthy living a compulsory and examinable subject, if they paid more attention to their students' posture and provided them with adjustable furniture to match their growth, they would produce healthier adults. That would take a big load off society for a start.

But it would not overcome one important factor, namely that from birth onwards the services are required of therapists who are not part of the medical system; therapists trained and experienced in palpatory and manipulative arts like midwives, osteopaths and chiropractors; those dedicated to enhancing health and relieving stress such as homoeopaths, naturopaths, yoga therapists, Alexander and Pilates teachers and acupuncturists; and above all integrated physicians who act as gatekeepers to refer patients to the optimum treatment, whatever their condition. All these today have to be paid for by the patient in addition to their taxes supporting inadequate national health systems and their insurance premiums. The disease clinics governments provide today should be supplemented by health clinics offering free osteopathic/chiropractic and naturopathic checkups every ten years for the whole nation (say around ages 1, 11, 21, 31 etc). The irony is that if all these modalities were included in national health systems, on an equal status to conventional medicine (as in Asia), the costs, the budgets and the risks to patients would be drastically reduced. The service would once more become sustainable.

And an end to backache!

Index

If you wish to order Dr Ali's *Integrated Health Bible*
simply telephone TBS Direct on 01206 255800